Reimagining the Body

REIMAGINING THE BODY

Somatic Practice, Embodiment, and the Science of Movement

Aline Newton
with Rebecca Carli-Mills

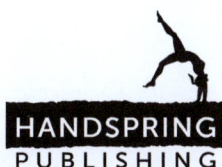

HANDSPRING
PUBLISHING

First published in Great Britain in 2026 by Handspring
Publishing, an imprint of Jessica Kingsley Publishers
Part of John Murray Press

1

A CIP catalogue record for this title is available from the
British Library and the Library of Congress

ISBN 978 1 80501 376 1
eISBN 978 1 80501 377 8

Printed and bound by CPI Group (UK) Ltd, Croydon, CR0 4YY

Jessica Kingsley Publishers' policy is to use papers that are natural,
renewable and recyclable products and made from wood grown in
sustainable forests. The logging and manufacturing processes are expected
to conform to the environmental regulations of the country of origin.

Handspring Publishing
Carmelite House
50 Victoria Embankment
London EC4Y 0DZ

www.handspringpublishing.com

John Murray Press
Part of Hodder & Stoughton Limited
An Hachette UK Company

The authorized representative in the EEA is Hachette Ireland, 8 Castlecourt
Centre, Dublin 15, D15 XTP3, Ireland (email: info@hbgi.ie)

Dedicated to Hubert Godard

with gratitude for his generosity and a lifetime of inspiration.

Contents

Acknowledgments

To produce a book is a team effort. I want to extend my deep appreciation to Rebecca Carli-Mills, friend and colleague for 38 years, without whom this book would not have been completed; to Karen D'Amato who was instrumental in working through many drafts; and to Jessica Kingsley Publishers for bringing the book into the world.

Hubert Godard's generosity with his teaching and time extended from the beginning of our studies in 1990. He freely allowed students to videotape workshops and to make transcripts and translations for our personal use. He continues to provide support through correspondence and meetings, culminating in the permission to use the material collected in this work.

Drafts of *Reimagining the Body* have been the required text in the three-semester Tonic Function Study Group taught with Rebecca since 2020. We would like to thank our students and colleagues for their valuable input.

To my friends and loved ones, human and four-legged, my family, and my partner, Peter Shapiro, thank you for all your contributions, feedback, and support, and for standing with me patiently over many years as the work took shape.

In addition, I would like to acknowledge the significant contributions of Dr. Ida P. Rolf, Michael Salveson, and Don Miller. Their wisdom, generosity, and approaches to practice have been essential to my own capacity to build a reliable sense of embodiment.

Orientation

HOW TO READ THIS BOOK

Gaston Bachelard writes: "The basic word in the lexicon of the imagination is not image, but imaginary" (Bachelard *et al.*, 2011, p.11). Instead of forming images, imagination offers the potential to change our perceptions, to allow us to experience something new.

In that spirit, *Reimagining the Body* offers an opportunity to free the body from the current tyranny of images—the body as a machine; the body as an object; the body split off from the mind, the brain, the computer, the executive; the body separated from our surroundings.

Instead of those limiting images, this book proposes constructive alternatives that lead to a richer experience of embodiment. By welcoming images from a surprising array of sources—from mobile robots to infants, from current neuroscientists to ancient Greeks—this book aims to provide readers with tools and confidence to aid in their own lifelong exploration of embodied intelligence.

Reimagining the Body provides a step-by-step guide through the landscape of embodiment, a path I have explored through 40 years of working with clients as a Rolfer® and somatic movement practitioner, 30 years of teaching, and decades of study with esteemed French Rolfer, somatic practitioner, dancer, and researcher, Hubert Godard, a highly influential leader in the overlapping communities of Rolfing®, Alexander, dance, and rehabilitative medicine. Based in years of clinical practice and teaching, Hubert Godard's approach to embodiment weaves many fields together—neuroscience, research, theory, and embodiment practices.

In this collaboratively completed edition, Rebecca Carli-Mills and I share with you the basis for an integrated perspective for embodiment practice based on research, client stories, and movement explorations developed over time and inspired by Hubert's teaching. Pseudonyms are used in client stories to protect privacy.

Embodiment is an inquiry that is ongoing by nature. Rather than arriving at a definition of embodiment, following the path of exploration put forward here will expand the dimensions of embodied experience available to the reader. The science of movement expands our imagination, while embodiment—experiential practices—brings theory to life, and workshop and client stories show the applications in a somatic practice.

BOOK ORGANIZATION

The book is organized into five parts.

Part I: Moving explores the tension between the standard mind/body images, their consequences for our sense of embodiment on the one hand, and, on the other, the research basis Hubert invited us to explore. Paradoxically, it is by turning to the history of mobile robots that we will be able to see human movement in the gravitational field more clearly. Each chapter includes experiential practices so that the consequences of the theory can be made clear through felt experience.

Part II: Expressing explores the negative impact the mind/body split can have and then offers an alternative framework that integrates the physical body with coordination, perception, and meaning. I share several experiences from workshops as well as client stories from my practice. The importance of orientation, perceptual choices, metaphors, and the physical basis of emotion are considered in depth.

Part III: Perceiving delves into body awareness, proprio- and interoception, kinesthesia, the role of gaze, and the kaleidoscope of interpretations of the concepts body schema and body image. Imagining is revealed as an inherent dimension of perception and emotion.

Part IV: Imagining presents a new imagining, recounting two embodiment practices that lead us into different experiences of self and introducing the term *action space* which includes our inherent relationship with our surroundings. The action space framework is followed into research and practice by presenting Hubert's research with breast cancer patients and a case study from my own practice in detail.

Part V: Becoming explores the early development of movement and emotional experience, when we are learning our body-in-the-world within the context of our caretakers. Understanding the roots of perception in the preverbal experience helps us approach change with clarity and courage.

Each of the five parts includes experiential opportunities (look for ✔) and embodiments: guided movement sequences; workshop scenarios, applications in practice (client stories), and supporting movement science. Images are accessed through QR codes. It is possible to follow any one of these threads as they spiral through all five sections, to read the book from cover to cover, or to take a non-linear approach. Many themes—our need for orientation in gravity, how we prepare for movement, the place of emotion, to name just a few—recur throughout the five parts. The book is also designed to be practiced and taken in slowly: each part takes a particular perspective on—a way of imagining—our embodied experience that represents years of study; and each practice benefits from repeated exploration and time.

Bachelard reminds us: "Thanks to the *imaginary*, imagination is essentially *open* and *elusive*. It is the human psyche's experience of *openness* and *novelty*." (Bachelard *et al.*, 2011, p.11) This is the body, reimagined.

Introduction

EMOTIONAL BODY

MEETING HUBERT

Hubert Godard had been teaching movement for 20 years when I first met him in 1990. On my bookshelves, magazine organizers full of notebooks testify to the numerous workshops I have taken with him over the years. On the off chance that I might have kept some notes from our first encounter, I take an organizer from the shelf. Remarkably, I find the material from that very first meeting: the 1990 Rolf Institute®[1] International Conference, when Rolfers from around the world gathered at the historic Boulderado Hotel on Pearl Street in Boulder, Colorado. The conference began with yoga, followed by the 10 a.m. keynote, to be given by "Hubert Godard, Rolfer and dancer." I had no idea who he was.

During the talk, Hubert showed a slide of Van Gogh's painting, "First Steps." [Figure 1] The painting shows a farmer in a field, his shovel on the ground beside him, and across the yard from the farmer—just beyond the garden's gate—a mother and toddler. The farmer crouches, offering his waiting arms to the child a few yards away; the little child stands with their mother's support and reaches towards the farmer.

How much there is in that moment! All the possibilities that emerge from getting up on two feet, the familiar presence of a mother who provides support, while the farmer's outstretched arms invite the child towards a great adventure: crossing the field. What will happen next? This is the story of standing up, the story of a living being who is always in relationship with physical surroundings, with human caregivers, and with gravity. In a sense, our relationship with gravity is the primary relationship: though an invisible presence, it is the most consistent force we experience.

Hubert explained that in order to move, we need first to be oriented in gravity—to know which way is up. Finding our way in gravity is an activity we are all engaging in as we stay upright and move, whether we realize it or not. Van Gogh's painting captures the moment when we take on our own independent management of gravity. Leaving the dependable support of the caregiver, we take a risk: we can lose our balance and fall over. Yet there are also benefits: we can explore the world on our own and develop agency. Working with gravity makes moving easy: a toddler toddles forward, going with the physical momentum. The farmer's waiting arms are an invitation and a reassurance: the child is drawn towards a safe harbor.

Figure 1: "First Steps"

Hubert described this interaction with gravity as the foundation of our earliest relationships and our own capacity for expression even before we stand or walk independently. This was a surprise to me: Hubert explained that even a newborn has already practiced movements in the womb, such as kicking faster or slower, arching and flexing, responding to different circumstances. These movements, called tonic, will become the foundation of postural support, and they also provide an infant with a channel of expression as they bicycle their legs in excitement or shrink away from too much stimulation (Bullinger, 2010). When met by an understanding caregiver, the movements become a form of communication.

As I listened to Hubert, "body in gravity" became more than a mechanical structure. Through his eyes, I could see us as body in motion, a meaning-filled expression, in which our physical experience, our relational experience, and our sense of self are all part of one system. He called this integrated perspective "tonic function." This was something I wanted to understand! It seemed like the perspective I had been seeking for many years. I knew right away that I wanted to study with Hubert Godard.

From our very first meeting, Hubert offered an alternative to the body/mind split, a different framework, in which a person is fundamentally in relationship with other people and our surroundings. But in addition, he offered a basis in neuroscience and research to ground the intuitions and give language to the experiences of practitioners in the field of somatics. This is the story that will unfold in the chapters that follow.

GETTING ROLFED

When I first met Dr. Ida P. Rolf, I was 11 years old, and she was an old lady with a flower in her white hair. My Uncle Mort had moved from New York City to California in the early 1960s and joined forces with a yoga guru, Richard Hittleman, when yoga was not nearly as mainstream as it is today. My uncle influenced my mother to take me to yoga classes while a small child, and through his connection with the Esalen Institute in Big Sur, California, he met Dr. Rolf, who was based in New York. When my grandmother had a mild stroke, Uncle Mort recommended she see Dr. Rolf. Then my grandmother told my mother to go see Dr. Rolf, and over time we became family friends with her sons and grandchildren. Little did I know then that this woman, known as *Grandma* affectionately to her students and officially to my playmates, would, through the power of her ideas, be a major influence on the course of my life and my choice of career. But at that time, in the early 1970s, Dr. Rolf was a presence at family dinners and, to me, just another grown-up.

Born in the Bronx in 1896, Dr. Rolf graduated from Barnard College in 1916 and had a rare opportunity for a woman at that time: to work at Rockefeller Institute (now Rockefeller University) while continuing her education. She went on to earn a Ph.D. in biological chemistry from the College of Physicians and Surgeons of Columbia University but left work in the late 1920s to take care of family matters. Over many years, she developed a technique of physical manipulation she called Structural Integration. By the 1950s, Dr. Rolf had developed the ten-session sequence of fascial manipulation known as the Rolfing series, based on the idea that a person's experience of health and ease—both physical and psychological—reflected the ease of that person's relationship with gravity, the most relentless force operating on us. While foundational for Rolfers for 75 years, to this day the effect of gravity in our daily movement continues to be a mostly unexplored factor and often goes unacknowledged outside the field.

In 1977, as I was finishing my first year of college, my uncle introduced my family to another Rolfer, Owen James. My parents suggested that I try a session, without specifying a particular reason. In his office, Owen looked at me and said: "I see a 17-year-old [my chronological age] and a four-year-old [the age of my past that I most identified with at the time] standing before me at the same time"—and this with hardly any conversation! How did he see what I was feeling?

The Rolfing session consisted of hands-on manipulation while I lay on a table or sat on a bench. In the course of the session, now and then I would get up, stand, or walk. To my surprise, with the physical work came many tears, but without a lot of thoughts or words. After the sessions, I found what I had considered psychological troubles—problems in my relationships, in my sense of self—almost magically transformed. I found myself able to respond more creatively to situations that would have upset me before. This was a big surprise for an analytically oriented young person, mired in the awkwardness and angst of late adolescence. It seemed that some of what I had considered emotional or behavioral patterns could be affected by working with the body, rather than just with words and ideas. This was the beginning of my understanding of "emotional body."

My Rolfing experience also challenged my understanding of "self." I could see that while talking about myself in therapy was speaking from an idea of myself, the hands-on work of Rolfing involved the sense of self itself. Today we might use a word like interoception to describe the emotional body, yet there was more to my experience than internal sensations. The physical changes through the Rolfing process led to changes in behavior. After my first few Rolfing sessions, I remember clearly feeling tongue-tied during a moment of conflict with a friend and finding myself with my weight on the outside edges of my foot. As I put my foot down, letting my whole foot rest on the ground, I was able to speak up for myself—putting my foot down, metaphorically, required a foot that could use the actual floor in action. These were my first experiences with the transforming emotion through the body in action. I became fascinated with the interaction of environment—the gravity field—body, and self or psyche. How could changing the relationship of the body in gravity result in changes in emotional patterns and action possibilities? I vowed to pursue Rolfing as a career, and a few years later, I began my training. Seven years later, I began my practice as a Certified Rolfer.

BLOCKS IN A BAG

In my first class at the Rolf Institute in 1984, I was introduced to Dr. Rolf's theories and practices. Dr. Rolf's work had come to prominence during the Human Potential Movement in the early 1970s. She was interested in transformation, in what allowed an individual full expression of themselves. She witnessed time after time how the process of Rolfing, which led to better alignment and relieved physical symptoms, also seemed to translate into a change—for the better—in how a person felt psychologically, something I had experienced myself. Dr. Rolf was a champion of gravity's importance for human beings. She wrote: "The gravitational field of the earth is easily the most potent physical influence in any human life. When human energy field and gravity are at war, needless to say gravity wins every time" (Rolf, 1977, p.30). In a world with gravity such as our own, if something—a pile of bricks, a building—is straight, lined up, then when gravity pulls down through the center, it will support the whole system. Conversely, when we are not using gravity with effective alignment, our joints suffer—gravity wins.

Dr. Rolf visualized the body in gravity as a stack of blocks. How are the major segments (head, chest, pelvis, legs) relating to each other? In this model, alignment looks like stacking up the blocks, so that gravity travels through an imaginary center line. Dr. Rolf envisioned the human being as a small energy field, not in an esoteric sense, but in material physical reality. "Symmetrical, balanced pattern" in the body's major segments would allow our lesser field to be reinforced by the greater field of the earth (Rolf, 1977, p.30). In other words, better alignment in gravity would translate into better physiological function for a person.

In Dr. Rolf's way of imagining, the stacked blocks were surrounded by a bag of fascia, connective tissue with an irregular arrangement of collagen fibers (Clemente, 1985; Standring, 2008). Fascia was significant because it was ubiquitous, continuous, and plastic—able to be changed. Dr. Rolf called the body's web of fascia the organ of structure or support (Rolf, 1977, p.37). She attributed the physical changes that people experienced through Rolfing to be an effect of the plasticity of connective tissue:

it could be freed from accumulated restrictions so that the body could regain optimal function. This was the Rolfer's mission.

Although she recognized its significance, Dr. Rolf saw gravity as a physical force affecting us from the outside, not accessible to an individual's experience. In her book, Dr. Rolf states unequivocally:

> Gravity is with us from the time of our conception to the moment of death. It is so all-pervading that we cannot sense it, for humans perceive sensory stimulation only as it varies. (We recognize light because there are periods of darkness, sound because we know quiet.) We do not sense gravity, but we do adjust to it. We must. (Rolf, 1977, p.31)

With the static image of alignment came an intuition of fascia as a moving, changing material that was at the root of the body's organization in relationship to gravity.

Rolfing manipulation could improve a person's function in gravity, but the task of organizing the body was left to the Rolfing practitioner. The client passively followed directions. In contrast, Hubert Godard, in his talk at the conference in 1990, invited us to discover our own *experience* of gravity. Rather than an external force, Hubert emphasized that being in relationship with gravity's force is an ongoing activity for each one of us, and as an ongoing experience, this is something we can affect. In each moment as we go about our day, with each step, each of us establishes a relationship with gravity as a support or as an impediment. This is something we can feel and befriend.

STACKING UP IN PRACTICE

In 1984, during my Rolfing training, we were asked to look at someone standing still and evaluate the person's alignment by seeing how far off the plumb line the different segments of their body lay. The structural metaphor "line the parts up and the body will work better in gravity" seemed tangible. Many approaches to body balance still find this useful: from our mothers' simple injunction to stand up straight, to ideas of alignment in some forms of dance, yoga, and tai chi. The connective tissue network, the fascial web, also remains an engaging image, as does seeing the body in relationship with gravity.

However, in my Rolfing practice, the goal of creating alignment produced mixed results. The structural metaphor seemed potentially measurable, but I found it difficult to apply to the person in front of me in my office. People felt better, but they did not end up straight. I found it problematic to ask someone to stand up straight, or to try to make points in the body line up (e.g., knees, ankles, and feet). For my clients, trying to keep their alignment often resulted in an artificial posture that was awkward and unsustainable. For a moment, people might show me their idealized image of good posture, but often, as soon as they moved, they would go back to their old way of standing. Imagining the body aligned from a static point of view did not translate into a living experience.

I also felt that something was missing from my initial training. Although deeply interesting, the theories about alignment and connective tissue did not help me understand my own experience of Rolfing: what led to the emotional experience and what changed my sense of myself, how I felt and behaved? Surprisingly to me, there was not much focus on this aspect when I first began my training as a Rolfer. The Rolfer's task was to deliver order in gravity to the client. The client's ongoing experience of this relationship was not part of the discussion. At the annual meeting six years later, to hear Hubert describe the importance of gravity from an experiential perspective, and to relate it to our emotional body and our relationship with other people, felt like such a welcome perspective—and much more true to my own experience. It seemed like what I had been waiting for.

BODIES MOVE!

Paradoxically, in spite of the insistence on the visual representation of the body's segments lining up, Dr. Rolf was fully aware of the power of movement. She practiced both yoga and tai chi into her senior years. This was a generative time in the U.S. when many of the somatic pioneers were crossing paths and influencing each other. Mabel Todd (1880–1956), F. M. Alexander (1869–1955), Moshe Feldenkrais (1904–1984), and Dr. Rolf (1896–1979) were all contemporaries and their perspectives intertwined.

Dr. Rolf was also fascinated by watching people in motion. Early in the 1950s, she befriended a dancer, Jennette Lee, who had been a student of F. M. Alexander. The story goes that Dr. Rolf and Ms. Lee went on long walks watching how people moved on the streets of New York City. Lee's approach to changing movement patterns included sensing weight as well as imagining releasing into the earth, and using the image of axes that radiate in all directions into the surrounding space to change the experience of movement (Lee, 1946). Though exposed to many practices and recognizing the power and significance of movement work for patients and for training Rolfing practitioners, Dr. Rolf never fully settled on a specific approach to movement.

In 1968, Dr. Rolf invited Judith Aston, a dancer who had found relief from injuries after working with Dr. Rolf, to develop a movement system that could accompany the Rolfing series. They worked together until 1977 before parting ways. Later, a series of other movement teachers further developed Rolf Movement Integration, each one bringing her own perspective, and the curriculum continued to evolve.

After my basic Rolfing training in 1984, in addition to movement workshops through the Rolf Institute, I continued to study a variety of approaches to movement: Iyengar yoga with Esther Meyers in Toronto where I lived at the time; an authentic movement tradition at the Centre of Movement with Leslie French. I studied qigong with Mantak Chia and Bruce Frantzis. I explored Feldenkrais work. But something was missing. We were instructed to do movements, often lying down, without much explanation. I didn't understand the "why." "It's the qi flow," "It's chakras," the teachers would say. If I asked too many questions, the teacher often got defensive. "You are too intellectual. Just learn through experience."

I never felt like I got it. None of the practices I learned had the impact of getting Rolfed, which had transformed my experience of life. No theory or practice made sense to me until I encountered Hubert Godard.

HUBERT'S STORY

Like Dr. Rolf, Hubert Godard started studying chemistry as a university student, but dance was his calling. Unfortunately, his body did not cooperate. Coming from a sports background, he didn't know better and forced his legs to turn out in what he thought was the ideal form required for classical ballet. By age 23, he had seriously damaged his knees. After an operation to repair a torn meniscus, he was unable to dance or even to walk without crutches for over a year and a half. Determined to find a way through this obstacle, he began to delve into anatomy, biomechanics, and movement analysis, exploring different approaches to movement and rehabilitation. Thus began his lifelong interest in rehabilitation techniques and research. Getting Rolfed during his exploration of differ-ent approaches to healing transformed Hubert's understanding of gravity. He said: "It is not the theory of Rolfing but being a client—I learned to rest."

Besides maintaining a Rolfing practice, Hubert was involved in teach-ing and research. A founder of Université Paris 8 Danse, he was influential in designing a program for dance education sponsored by the French government to protect young dancers from injury. He also worked with musicians, running a movement laboratory with the National Orchestra in Liège, Belgium. In addition, Hubert conducted research at the National Cancer Institute in Milan, Italy, where he worked with the doctors on their own embodiment and to individualize breast cancer rehabilitation. He brought all this experience to teaching about movement.

STUDIES WITH HUBERT

I had been a Rolfer for six years when I met Hubert. At the 1990 confer-ence in Boulder, Hubert held a workshop that introduced participants to his approach to movement based on his synthesis of dance, Alexander Technique, Mezières Method,[2] and Rolfing work. Instead of a static image of alignment to describe organization in gravity, Hubert talked about *ori-enting* in gravity. He described a line that went in two directions: towards the heavens and into the earth, an activity without end.

Introducing G'

At the workshop, Hubert invited us to pick up a rolled-up blanket as if we were picking up a baby—"to change G'." A common definition of the cen-ter of gravity, G, is the imaginary point of balance where the body's weight is concentrated. For a human body, the rule of thumb is somewhere below the belly button in the middle of the lower trunk. But Hubert introduced us to the idea of G': a secondary, or partial, center of gravity, the center of gravity of the chest, arms, and head, located just in front of the fourth thoracic vertebra (T4). Seen in motion in reference to an imaginary line running between the heads of the two femurs (the trans-coxo-femoral axis), the freedom of movement of G' impacts the mechanics of the whole movement (Sohier & Haye, 1989). Looking at a center of gravity of the trunk and upper body as we go into movement? This was new! The impor-tance of G' was a revelation.

In the same workshop, Hubert gave us each a little marionette on a string. Following his instructions, I held the marionette by the string with an outstretched arm in front of my chest and ran across the room, stopping periodically and trying not to let the marionette swing. The marionette acted like a biofeedback device: if G' was held too stiffly, the force of the sudden stop would be transferred to the marionette. These movement practices sensitized us to a new aspect of organizing our movement in gravity.

EMBODIMENT: WAITING TO BE CALLED

In another exercise, Hubert asked to borrow small belongings from participants: a jacket, a bag, a book. He placed them in the middle of the circle of seated participants, not too far from each other. He then asked a volunteer to "pick up the objects one by one and put them back." After the volunteer had done so, Hubert asked that they do it again, "but this time wait for the jacket to call your hand." As we watched our classmate, it seemed that waiting a moment before beginning to reach translated into a slight release in the arm and a more graceful gesture. Taking a different starting point brought a change in the quality of the movement: there was listening here. When I tried it myself, I felt the change in attitude and a shift in the action itself. Instead of tightening my hand around the jacket, there was breathing room, a sense of spaciousness in the contact. "And now wait for the floor to call the jacket before putting it back," Hubert said. I could feel the difference as I paused to wait for the earth's pull, though I did not yet have language to describe or explain the experience. Such a simple exercise! To interact with objects is something we do every day. We put down our coffee cup, we pick up our pen; getting dressed is a series of movements of reaching and letting go. The simple change that Hubert suggested took these movements from mundane and unconscious actions and transformed the world into call and response, a constant being-in-relation. The mundane action became a poetic gesture, while also improving from a biomechanical perspective: we used less effort and created less compression in our joints as we moved through the actions. It is its very simplicity that makes this practice hard to remember with every breath and every gesture.

From that very first meeting came the seeds that grew over the course of several decades into the perspective described in detail in this book, in which we are not separate from our surroundings, in which movement, imagination, emotion, and perception can be addressed as a dynamic whole.

CHALLENGING ASSUMPTIONS

Following the meeting in 1990, my colleagues and I felt an urgency to organize workshops with Hubert so we could continue to learn. We would meet intensively for five or six days in Boulder, Berkeley, or Philadelphia, Holderness, NH, Paris, Munich, or Rome—but always in a dance studio or hall, spacious but often without mirrors. We would always begin sitting in a circle on chairs, around 15 of us. We introduced ourselves, saying if we had an injury or physical problem, or if we had particular questions or interests. Then Hubert would begin to talk at a breakneck pace. A Renaissance man of movement, Hubert's work was on the leading edge of the revolution in neuroscience that has been taking place since the early 1990s. He would bring us papers to read, and he would help us understand why the information was important. The workshops were a focal point during which research and concepts were introduced that gave a background to the embodiment practices we were experiencing. Over many years, meeting at workshops provided an opportunity to develop our understanding of recent neuroscientific discoveries through conversation in a collegial atmosphere. We were then able to take these practices and concepts into further study in our professional practices with our clients. The goal of this book is to share the workshops with you, elaborating the concepts and the practices, so you too can arrive at a reimagining of the body.

Some of the research studies Hubert introduced to us highlighted puzzling aspects of movement that challenged our conventional understanding of intention and awareness. For instance, British neuropsychologist Lawrence Weiskrantz (1926–2018) coined the term *blindsight* to describe a form of blindness in which the eye itself is not affected—the retinas are intact—yet the person still reports that they cannot see (Weiskrantz *et al.*, 1974). Despite this, in studies, blindsighted individuals successfully navigated a hallway crowded with obstacles, and could spontaneously reorient a letter to fit through a mail slot, all the while maintaining that they could not see. The blindsight studies were intriguing: if the patients could not see, what sense were they using to navigate their environments? If not their conscious minds, what part of them was managing their movements in relation to their surroundings?

Similarly, the neuroscientist V. S. Ramachandran's studies on phantom limb pain challenged my understanding of the mind/body relationship. In one experiment, a subject who had an arm amputation had phantom limb pain as well as experiencing the phantom limb as paralyzed. The very existence of phantom limbs brings up questions: the brain is making a map of a body which is not the actual body. How does the brain imagine a limb that isn't there, let alone a limb that isn't there but is painful and paralyzed? But Ramachandran also wanted to find a remedy for the problem. He came up with the idea of the mirror-box: an open box into which each arm could be inserted. [Figure 2] Ramachandran positioned the subject in front of this device. The mirror inside the box reflected the patient's actual arm, creating the illusion that it was located on the amputated side. Ramachandran then asked the subject to move the actual arm. In the reflection, the amputated arm had reappeared and was moving. Remarkably, this visual representation caused both the paralysis of the phantom limb and the pain associated with it to disappear (Ramachandran, 1994). What did this mean about how our brain locates our body? Ramachandran's research challenges standard views of the brain as a computer with clear pathways and modular components. Instead, it suggests that our model of reality may not be as stable as we imagine. How would this change our approach to movement practice and healing?

Figure 2: Ramachandran's mirror box

In a third example, Hubert's own work with breast cancer patients challenged our understanding of muscle function. With funding from the Italian government, he was part of a team studying how to choose the best muscle for breast reconstruction. He explained that the decision had originally been based on the patient's body size: for larger women, the surgeons generally chose rectus abdominis, and for smaller women, latissimus dorsi. But the results were not satisfying: secondary problems often arose after the surgery.

Hubert and his colleagues found that in some women, the removal of latissimus dorsi had no ill effect, while in other women, it led to a kind of collapse in the structure. The effect of removing either muscle depended on how the individual woman used that muscle, what Hubert called "her postural signature or coordination," her way of organizing herself in gravity.

Anatomy books present charts of muscle action that always start from the same anatomical position. But in real life, the context matters. Hubert's research had shown him that the function of a given muscle depended on how a woman organized her uprightness. Some people might use latissimus dorsi as a key muscle in their postural organization, while for others it might not be central to this overall coordination. The impact of removing a particular muscle would depend on the individual's particular strategy for staying upright. This is a different vision from Dr. Rolf's passive blocks in a bag, while still describing a person's relationship to gravity. In the 1990s, this new perspective that considered individual postural strategy allowed for more effective choices in breast reconstruction surgery. Thirty years later, we now have research on individuals' unique movement signatures that supports Hubert's perspective (Hug *et al.*, 2019).

Hubert's insights were based on his experience with patients and working with his own body, while also drawing on a rich vein of research from movement and perception scientists such as James Gibson, Nikolai Bernstein, and Esther Thelen. We will explore their contributions in the chapters ahead. Hubert's ease and joy in exploring research connected us as practitioners to a large and interesting field of scientific inquiry that can nourish somatic practice. Although many of the pioneers of somatic traditions have passed away, the new research confirms many of their ideas and clarifies others. After presenting these mind-blowing new perspectives from current research, we would move on to a movement practice—"embodiment." Hubert would call it—that helped us connect the theory with a felt experience.

EMBODIMENT: STICK WORK, AN APPROACH TO CORE COMPETENCE

The vignette that is described in this section is an example of what Hubert called "embodiment"—the part of our workshops in which we explored our lived experience while Hubert directed our attention in various ways. As in *Waiting to be called*, described earlier in this chapter, often we would use an object as part of the experience. Borrowing the pediatrician and psychoanalyst Donald Winnicott's (1896–1971) term, Hubert called these objects "transitional objects." For a young child, a transitional object is "the first 'not-me' possession" (Winnicott, 1953, p.5). In Hubert's approach to movement, the transitional object allows us to be in relationship with an Other, instead of being self-focused as we move. This way, an embodiment practice could include exploring our biomechanics in gravity while also exploring how our relationship to our surroundings and other people impacts our movement systems. In this embodiment practice, each class member was given a wooden stick about the size of a closet dowel. The practice evolved our experience of "core."

We stood, holding the stick in both hands with our arms hanging in front of us at ease. Hubert began to direct us: "First, let yourself notice where you and the stick are touching. Notice the place of contact—it is a two-way process: you are touching the stick and being touched by the stick at the same time."

It was a simple invitation and obviously literally true, but the effect was surprising. As my hands touched the stick, felt the stick, and allowed the stick to rest into my fingers and palms as if the stick too was animate, somehow gripping the stick felt different. A kind of tension in my hands let go, as I shifted my perception to feeling the stick touching me.

How is this possible? I wondered. But the actual experience was clear. Hubert explained that when I shifted to the perception of "being touched by the stick," on a muscular level the bigger forearm muscles released, making way for the muscles local to the hand and palm itself to work first. What was surprising to me was that a change in how I was paying attention, or how I described my action to myself—how I imagined it— could change the motor pattern. To my surprise, almost simultaneously, I felt a sense of engagement in the belly wall, one that did not feel like a sit-up or pulling the chest closer to the hips and pelvis but that provided an increase in stability around the spine. It seemed to happen of its own accord in response to the change to the sense of being touched.

The standard definition of core muscles is that they are abdominal mus-cles that we work out to strengthen, but in this case, the feeling of stability came with no deliberate effort; the organization of support of the lumbar spine came of its own in response to letting myself feel the touch of the stick.[3]

Hubert continued: "Even your palms have something to do with the 'core muscles.' Core muscles are not the same as abdominal muscles. It is a way your brain helps keep you stable, or perhaps more poetically, it is how you manage instability. It's the contact with the object, with the world, through your hands and feet that triggers it." Instead of focusing on will-power and voluntary muscular contraction, we changed our attitude. Our practice with the stick was strengthening to the body, but it also included a sense of meaningfulness: touching and being touched, a way of meeting many facets of our daily life. Hubert was inviting us into a new way of seeing, feeling, and working in movement, where the physical dimension of muscle activation felt effortless and was inseparable from the emotional experience of being in relationship.

For me, this was radical: to understand core as a function related to how I stayed stable, and how I stayed stable was directly affected by how I engaged with my surroundings—in this case, the stick. This quality of core stability is evoked when we encounter our world, finding the appro-priate balance between touching and being touched in any given moment (Merleau-Ponty, 1964).

"Now," Hubert continued, "let the stick begin to…as if float up…and let your hands follow it." Though a simple invitation, the movement was entirely different than when I set my intention to lift the stick myself. While my imagination *was* being exercised, there was no sense of physical effort. "Imagine it is lifting up and you are hanging from it." How is it possible that I feel as if I am hanging from a stick that I am clearly holding up in the air? What is different, what has changed?

Hubert went on: "Now the stick is becoming a heavy weight, pulling you over into a forward bend. Now coming up still with a sense of the stick as heavy, you can feel each pair of vertebrae link into a system as you stand up." Hubert continued: "Instead of using the big muscles of hips and shoulders, you are activating the postural muscles, the ones in a better position to work to support the bony skeleton without getting in the way of freedom to move."

These familiar exercises from yoga or a stretching routine now made a different kind of sense. I was fascinated. In other movement disciplines, I found myself going through the motions, as the saying goes. None of the explanations had satisfied me, and the admonishment to "just do it and then you will understand" had not been satisfying either. I wanted to understand why: what was the point of what I was doing? I needed words and concepts to orient me to movement practices, and movement practices to help me embody the big ideas. Guided by Hubert, the movement was not about piecemeal strengthening of muscles nor was it about flexibility per se. Yet it had a huge effect: it was a practice of being with, being here, that led to a change that was physical and emotional simultaneously.

In daily life, movements have meaning—they are purposeful. We may be trying to accomplish something, such as lifting a grocery bag, or to express something, like opening our arms to hug someone. But most of the time in exercise classes we are asked to do movements—such as raising our arms—with no relationship to their meaning. Our practice with the stick was not a simple pragmatic action, but instead invited a different experience in movement: a relationship. It isn't the stick itself that matters. The movements included the meaning that touching and being touched had for each one of us. From the very first classes, Hubert's teaching changed my understanding of exercise from an attempt to master to a change in relationship with the world and objects around me.

As with the embodiment practices described in each chapter throughout this book, you can try this for yourself.

TRY THIS   ↓

For instance, when reaching for your phone or your coffee cup, feel the difference between the action of grasping the phone—me grasping—and the action of letting the phone rest in your palm, feeling its weight. Can you sense a shift in the tension in your arms or hand?

To switch to feeling the phone touching you, your brain chooses a different way of moving—a different neuromuscular pathway—and a different attitude toward the world.

Over the next three decades, Hubert would share with us an evolving conceptual framework along with embodiment practices that the other students and I felt the effects of in our lives—practically, personally, and professionally. The theory and the practices always situated us in our gravitational context and our context as human meaning makers, working with orientation and perception and imagination.

PART I

MOVING

CHAPTER ONE

Mechanical Body

How did I end up turning to artificial intelligence and mobile robots to make sense of human movement? From 1990 onward, I continued to study with Hubert whenever I could. The workshops I attended were for Rolfers who already had a common language and base of experience, but I wanted to share my growing understanding in a wider field.

After more than a decade of study with Hubert, in 2004 an opportunity came my way to collaborate with the MIT gymnastics coach, Noah Riskin. As a gymnast, Noah had first-hand experience of his body's intelligence as a moving and balancing system. He had devised a playful class for the January inter-session in which students would experience some aspects of what he was calling physical intelligence through elaborate falling competitions and other games. After we were introduced by a Rolfing client of mine who detected our common interests, Noah and I began to collaborate on a more complex course using experiential learning techniques supported by the research information I had been following under Hubert's direction. For example, Hubert's research with breast cancer patients reinforced Dr. Rolf's perspective that how we organize ourselves in gravity was a very important aspect of every movement. Weiskrantz's research on blindsight suggested that there was more than just our conscious intention helping us navigate when we move through space, while Ramachandran's phantom limbs implied that our brains are engaged in a process of invention about exactly what constitutes "my body." These puzzles were clues to ways of working with ourselves as moving systems with physical intelligence. Yet all this stood in contrast to the standard view of movement health that consists primarily of voluntary muscular contraction through repetitive exercise of individual muscle groups. How could we help our students bridge this gap?

MIT CLASS

The course syllabus presented the body as "the very basis of our experience in the world" and "the very foundation on which cognitive intelligence is built." Together, Noah and I came up with a curriculum based on our combined experiences of Rolfing and gymnastics. While we originally conceived of the Physical Intelligence project as a course of study that would begin freshman year and build through the four years of college, funding was only given for a one-semester pilot-project class for seniors in the engineering department—PE for MEs, or Physical Education for Mechanical Engineers. It would be taught in the last semester before graduation, and participants would be tasked with designing a product based on the "physical intelligence" principles that we presented. We were asking them to discover a whole new way of understanding bodies and movement, and to come up with a product they would design and build—in just 14 weeks. And graduating depended on it!

How could I get through to these engineering students that the body isn't a thing but an organism? That the organism has its own intelligence? How could I convey what it actually means to be "organizing ourselves in gravity"? We made a valiant attempt that ultimately resulted in several products and patents. In one of the more successful class sessions, we used the ropes course in the MIT gymnasium so each student could experience for themselves the sensations associated with terror or exhilaration as they climbed up to the flying trapeze, strapped in for safety, and let go to swing across the length of the gymnasium. The experience was completely controlled but made the point that our emotions are sensory experiences and not just in our heads.

However, I sensed that none of the areas that appealed to me in Hubert's way of working—philosophy, phenomenology, depth psychology, even something as simple and practical as finding more ease in movement—felt compelling for our students. Noah and I were looking for a field trip to inspire them, something dynamic, when I came across the MIT museum's exhibit on the history of artificial intelligence and its current developments. I thought the engineers would appreciate the irony: at MIT, the phrase "embodied intelligence" referred to robotics. Unexpectedly, exploring the history of mobile robots turned out to be a great way to make sense of human movement, to bring in some of the missing pieces between the standard view of the body and what I had learned from years of studying with Hubert. In this chapter, I will share some examples from the MIT museum's exhibit in order to explore what building mobile robots reveals about how we humans manage the complex work of getting around.

EMBODIED INTELLIGENCE

Hubert used the term "embodiment" to name the movement practices that linked a concept with a felt experience. But the term was also used in a different context: to describe a hot topic for hardcore scientists working in the field of artificial intelligence. What did this term mean to them? Artificial intelligence encompasses many lines of research. Most people are familiar with the latest large language models known as chatbots. But another field of inquiry has been developing in research circles in which scientists turn to animals and insects, to biological systems, to gain insights into the ingenious processes that go into living as a body. One approach is to try to build a system that can do some of the behaviors observed in organic systems. The engineers call it "understanding by building." Looking into the work of the engineers trying to make creatures that can move independently brought to light many important aspects of human movement that we normally take for granted.

Usually when I mention embodiment and robotics in conversation ("Oh, you're writing a book? What is it about?"), people often conclude that computer scientists have discovered once and for all that we don't need our bodies—that the body is unnecessary. In fact, it's quite the contrary. Early 21st-century artificial intelligence systems were wildly successful at challenges such as chess but failed miserably at behaviors like seeing or walking that we may take for granted. What was missing? The roboticists began to wonder if moving in an environment might be the key. What if intelligence arose from the interaction between a system and its environment? In trying to make a robot that can move independently in the world, roboticists have developed an appreciation for just how significant it is to be a body. For the MIT engineers in our class, learning what is involved in building a mobile robot gave them a better appreciation for their own amazing systems.

It is unsurprising that people jump to the conclusion that the body is unnecessary. It reflects a common worldview: the body is the car; the mind is the driver. When my friend Auren was only 11, he told me of a book he had read called *The Six* (Alpert, 2016). It tells the story of a terminally ill child with muscular dystrophy whose father figures out how to transfer the boy's brain signals into a robot. Although the body would die, the child would live on in the robot body—and not only that. In the story, the child's "signature" (the collection of brain signals) could be transferred in and out of all kinds of machines at will. In *The Six*, the body is completely irrelevant, and we can live forever! I can see the appeal of this point of view. The author, Mark Alpert, an editor at *Scientific American*, wanted to introduce young people to the wonders of science. He claimed his novel "isn't science fiction" (Alpert, n.d.).

Alpert's view reflects a prevalent cultural attitude. Societally, we imagine ourselves as singularly dissociated from our surroundings, often disembodied and growing more so daily. We rarely give importance to where we actually are. It is a given and our minds are elsewhere: dwelling on yesterday's troubles, anticipating tomorrow's events, or surfing the web, the disembodied experience par excellence. To concentrate, we try to tune out most of the sounds (distractions) in the environment with the aid of headsets, and we learn to disregard the signals from our body-self almost entirely to live in the space between our eyes and the screen. On Zoom meetings, we create our own virtual surroundings; we can set our backdrop to whatever scene pleases us. Disembodied, like the children in *The Six*, we could be anywhere, all the power in our minds alone.

SOME*WHERE*

Not so fast, says Alan Jasanoff, an MIT neuroscientist/engineer. In his book *Biological Mind* (2018), he dubs attitudes like Alpert's, the "cerebral mystique." Jasanoff critiques the common images of the brain as a computer. A brain that can be separated from the body, independently controlling our intentions and actions, is a fantasy. This fantasy perpetuates a false impression of the brain as the executive and the body as a replaceable laborer. The false image also completely disregards our essential relationship to our environment.

When we come back to reality, we understand that certain things follow from being a body—things so obvious they are often overlooked. As a body, we are always embedded in a particular environment, situated. One of the requirements of embodiment (meaning, in this case, just living as a body) is to be *somewhere*; a body is located somewhere specific. This may seem trivial, but think for just a moment: what does it mean to be "here"? It's not just mindfulness! "Here" means that we are interacting with forces in the environment, like gravity. "Here" also requires moving, getting around. Successful organisms evolve in partnership with a specific environment, so that moving can be energy efficient—or they wouldn't be able to survive. In our rapidly evolving artificial environments, we have lost sight of this partnership.

TRY THIS

Tune in to the surfaces of your body in contact with your chair or, if standing, the soles of your feet touching the ground. Notice the places of contact... Scan to find them all.

Gently guide your attention to notice that the chair and ground are also touching you: your back, legs, pelvis, and feet... Shift your awareness to receive this touch. Take a few moments to build two-directional awareness—you are touching, but you are also being touched...

You might have the instinct to move more fully into the touch so that there is a felt sense of a meeting. You might notice changes in your breathing, heart rate, or felt state...

Now, slightly shift your focus to become aware of the whole of your environment—the space around, behind, and above you. You may notice the ambient sounds in your space...

Perhaps you find yourself wishing to change position in response to this process of orienting to where you are right now. If so, gently shift in response...

ROBOTIC TUNA: EFFORTLESS ACTION AND ENVIRONMENT

A robotic tuna displayed at the MIT museum compellingly illustrated the important connection between where we are and how we move. [Figure 3] Robotuna was designed for studying underwater propulsion in an attempt to build better submarines. The four-foot-long robot had a sleek, streamlined shape, resembling an Atlantic bluefin tuna: "2,843 parts include over 40 ribs, a set of tendons, a segmented backbone with vertebrae and, of course, its Lycra skin" (MIT News, 1994). This early version of the robofish was connected to a mechanical structure that housed the electronics and guided it in the testing tank in the basement of MIT.

By designing and building a mechanical version of a tuna, MIT scientists in the laboratory of Michael Triantafyllou were able to figure out how the tuna achieves its powerful, efficient swimming. The secret is jet propulsion. To get around in the ocean, the tuna's large vertical tail flicks the water to one side, forming a spinning vortex, and to the other side, forming another vortex. When the two vortices combine behind the tuna, they create jet propulsion—the water pushes the tuna. The tuna is not *pulling* itself through the water, struggling and straining. Instead, the tuna mobilizes the forces available in the environment to do the work. This example of brilliant adaptation makes the tuna one of the ocean's top swimmers (Triantafyllou & Triantafyllou, 1995).

Robotuna was a successful experiment—more efficient and more maneuverable than previous robotic submarines, and it was a success for the mechanical engineers in the class too: it provided an analogy that they could connect with! Moving—what mobile organisms need to do to feed and escape from predators among other essential activities—has to be efficient. Whether we call it exploiting the forces provided by the environment or evolving in sync with our environment, all organisms are adapted to move in a particular milieu. Surroundings matter. How does this apply to human beings?

Figure 3: Robotuna

In theory, humans have evolved to navigate our "ocean"—the field of gravity—as skillfully and efficiently as the tuna swims in the sea (Gracovetsky, 1988). The connective tissues of the human body, our "organ of support"—Dr. Rolf's web of fascia—is elastic (Rolf, 1977, p.37). As we take a step, this elasticity can allow us to extend, which stores kinetic energy in the gravitational field. With each step we take, we can potentially use that kinetic energy to propel our next step. Our weight meeting the ground is a force: in physics terms, the force provokes an equal and opposite response. Elastic tissues and ground forces can make walking feel nearly effortless. This makes sense when we remember that we are organisms: a low expenditure of energy just to get from here to there is crucial to survival.

As we'll see later, walking is a great way for bipeds with spines like ours to use the gravitational field of this planet. On a planet with lesser gravitational pull, we might have evolved to hop instead. On the space station, for example, astronauts get around using swimming movements. Without the force of gravity, they must exercise to keep their bones from disintegrating. Our most basic body structure, our very shape, is part of being here on this planet.

Unfortunately, people rarely experience moving as effortless. Unlike the tuna and most of our distant ancestors, the efficiency of our movement is no longer the key to our survival. Yet, while our lives may not seem to be immediately at stake, over the long run, we pay for our inefficiency in tension, lack of energy, bad posture, and bad moods as well as joint injury and pain.

Without the constraint of survival, we are "free" to move without regard for maximum efficiency—for better or worse. The mechanical engineers in my class at MIT were young athletes who spent a lot of time sitting in school. They probably suffered from having too much energy rather than feeling the need to conserve it. They were also young enough not to notice the effects of working against gravity instead of with it.

Working with gravity for more efficient movement is more than just a matter of being faster than the other guy; it is also a likely contributor to our long-term health. The ease of each and every breath depends on the coordination that keeps us from falling over as inhaling and exhaling change our balance point; good organization in gravity allows the most freedom for breath, affecting our mental and emotional state. Good organization in gravity—the proper tone without excess tension—provides the best environment for our organ systems to operate, for digestion, for vitality. Half a century after Dr. Rolf pointed it out, effective use of the gravitational field is still mostly not considered an aspect of our health.

In our day and age, and perhaps especially in the US, we have instead turned effort into a positive ethic. "No pain, no gain," children hear in gym class, as adults do from personal trainers. But the robotic tuna shows us something different, something surprisingly closer to what Hubert taught me. As it mobilizes the water to create jet propulsion, it is more like a qi master, at one with the environment in which it is embedded. It is ironic that a robotic tuna designed by an MIT engineer provided an up-to-date example for my students of a very old concept: the mysterious paradox of *wei wu wei*, action without action, sometimes called non-doing. Far from an esoteric Eastern ideal, this idea could translate into letting the organism do what it does well without our interference. How would we go about it?

ECOLOGICAL PSYCHOLOGY

To understand more deeply how the essential relationship between living creatures and their environment impacts their movement, Hubert turned us towards the work of James J. Gibson (1904–1979), an accomplished cognitive psychologist who studied perception. Gibson became famous during World War II through his work to identify the visual information required for a pilot to safely land an airplane.

By observing and interviewing pilots, he discovered that much of the crucial information they used for landing came directly from the visual environment, rather than from internal calculations or solely from cockpit instruments.

Prior to Gibson's work, many researchers assumed that perception involved the brain constructing detailed internal images or mental models of the world. The prevailing idea was that pilots had to do a kind of mental math of size, distance, and speed to guide their approach. Gibson's discovery suggested a more direct form of perception: the visual patterns or "flows" of light coming from the runway, the horizon, and surrounding terrain offered immediate information about the plane's movement and orientation. Gibson noted that as a pilot approaches the runway, the pattern of the ground surface texture (like fields or the runway lights) expands outward from a point directly ahead. This "optic flow" signals changes in altitude and angle of descent, allowing a pilot to adjust approach and speed without mentally computing distance or angles. Instead of relying on internal estimates or memory, pilots could simply "read" the environment. This direct perception theory was a departure from the idea that the mind must first process and interpret raw sensations before producing a perceptual understanding.

The new and unusual aspect of Gibson's discovery lay in showing that perception—especially in a high-stakes, real-world activity like landing a plane—depends on detecting structured patterns in the environment itself. This helped lay the groundwork for his "ecological approach" to perception, emphasizing that the visual world provides rich, ready-made information essential for successful action.

Gibson's work challenged the status quo of stimulus–response psychological research in which passive subjects were exposed to a stimulus and their responses studied. Gibson felt that to understand perception, we needed to consider animals as *active* agents: how we orient, how we select meaningful information from our environment, how we keep in touch with our world (Reed, 1988).

A committed experimentalist and theorist, Gibson wanted to reframe the basic questions of psychology. The key question was: "How do animals (including humans) respond to their environment?" Perception was "not based on having sensations," Gibson wrote, "but it is surely based on detecting information" (Gibson, 1966, p.2). By "information," Gibson referred to the energy of light, touch, and sound that comes to us as structures or patterns detectable by an animal and, above all, useful for navigating. In the terrestrial environment, gravity is another information source as we use it every breath and every step to maintain our balance.[1]

Gibson described what an animal perceives as the affordances in the environment, the resources or functional properties of places or things that are relevant or meaningful.

Affordances are opportunities for action that we can directly perceive without the need for complex mental interpretation. An affordance is not just a property of an object; it is a relationship between the object's features and the abilities of the individual looking at it. For a person, an apple affords eating, baking into a pie, throwing. For a worm, it could be a food supply or a house. Something can be an affordance only if it suits the abilities and needs of whoever encounters it.

In reframing our relationship with our environment in this way, Gibson was attempting to get away from the tradition of dualistic thinking—for example, subject/object, self/environment—that he felt plagued psychology. He wanted to escape from the inheritance of philosopher Descartes (1596–1650) which split physical or primary qualities, the stimuli, from secondary or psychological qualities, the results of the stimuli, our responses. According to Gibson, animate and aware creatures perceive themselves in the world, not separated from it. He called his approach "ecological psychology." To this day, it is considered one of the major theories describing how we move (Shumway-Cook *et al.*, 2024).

Gibson was successful in his time. His standing afforded him the security to be outspoken and somewhat controversial. He was a professor of experimental psychology at Smith College during the Depression. From his position at Cornell from the early 1950s onward, he was elected to the National Academy of Sciences in 1967 and received a Senior Career Development Award from the National Institute of Mental Health, which supported his work through the end of his life.

Gibson's variables—orienting, perception, and action, how we select and pick up useful information from the environment—were the same ones that arose in working with movement in workshops, in our sessions with clients, and in life. His point of view provided us with a link between Dr. Rolf's recognition of the power of gravity in human function—a good example of useful information provided by the environment—Hubert's approach to movement work which invited us to pay attention to this useful information, and a range of academic disciplines. Scientists are reevaluating the notion that the way to understand our behavior is by breaking it down into ever simpler parts, or seeking the answers in a computationally marvelous, disembodied brain. From rehab to robotics, Gibson's work provides contemporary researchers with an alternative to the cerebral mystique that is so prevalent in our culture today.

IN CONTEXT: ROBOROACH DISPELS THE CEREBRAL MYSTIQUE

It was a joyful irony that the robot designs we saw at the MIT museum helped me make a case to the mechanical engineers in my class that movement is a complex, non-linear behavior that cannot be understood in a traditional top-down model. As we will see with the next exhibit, Roboroach, that model did not work to build a mobile robot, and it doesn't work for us. Instead, Hubert's approach to movement work and the robotics exhibits at the MIT museum were considering body, brain, and the environment together in order to understand how we move.

Of all creatures, the cockroach is recognized as an amazing climber. Its six legs help it navigate difficult terrain and easily make its way over obstacles—perfect skills for a robot. The next exhibit at the MIT museum was indeed a robotic cockroach: Roboroach. [Figure 4] The scientists and engineers who created Roboroach started with pure mechanics to unlock the mystery of the cockroach's skill: they carefully measured all the joints to make a blueprint. Then they built their model to those specifications.

In this construction, wires took the place of the nerve signals to the muscles which are considered the "engines of movement." Roboroach was interesting to look at, with its metallic frame, jointed legs, and pistons, significantly larger than an actual roach, but it could not move, let alone climb. The machine could not even stand up. To the researchers' surprise, building an accurate structure with muscle "engines" was not enough. All those movable joints did not result in effective movement. The robotic tuna and robotic cockroach got the engineering students thinking along the same lines as Gibson: how does the cockroach get around, navigate its environment, and what makes it such a successful climber?

Figure 4: Roboroach

Initially, the robotics researchers thought about the cockroach's movement the same way you or I might: the whole is the sum of the parts. To build a system that could move, they started by building the structure as it appeared at a standstill. Nice and simple. They also approached controlling movement in a simple, linear way: as if the brain controls each muscle, telling each one what to do. In this classic model of movement, we imagine a top-down hierarchy with the brain as the boss (the "computer"). Of course, so far, we do seem to need our brains, but the failure of early versions of the Roboroach shows that the model in which the brain tells each muscle what to do does not produce complex, functional movement.

Dr. Rolf attributed one of her favorite sayings to Alfred Korzybksi[2]—"If you want a different conclusion, start with a different premise" (Feitis, 1978, p.42). The mystery of the cockroach's movement was solved when the researchers started to envision moving in a non-linear way, from a systems perspective. Instead of trying to understand the system by separating it into components, they started to look at the bigger picture: how the parts cooperate to produce the roach's behavior. In this case, they began to consider the cockroach's climbing ability as *an activity that includes the environment.* Instead of structures and individual muscle engines, they looked at how the cockroach's legs work together with the ground.

Each of the three pairs of legs has a particular role: the middle pair of legs keeps the insect stable, while the back pair pushes off the ground and the front pair reaches. Stabilizing, reaching, and pushing are how the cockroach manages the forces the environment presents. The coordination of the pairs of legs, the sequence and timing of the movement, all serve the cockroach's needs in the world: climbing to explore or survive. Rather than seeking the key to movement in the parts, the researchers succeeded in imitating the roach's movements by looking at the way a movement is organized as an interaction with place—how the cockroach's legs worked with the ground and in service of the actions necessary for getting around in the world—brain, body, and environment together. In the process of building a machine that can actually move, robotics researchers are helping create a different image of being embodied—one in which body and world move in an ongoing dance.

Materials management

The next exhibit at the MIT museum showed a video of a pair of linked robotic legs walking down a ramp. In another testament against the cerebral mystique, no brain was needed for this movement, just lower limbs and the angle of the ramp. Something similar would be true for you and me: as human beings, our movements are influenced by their context much more than we assume. For example, in the loop I run around the pond in my neighborhood, the path is fairly level until about halfway, and then it begins to slope downhill. At that point, I start running faster without trying. Gravity speeds up my body and my legs have to move faster. Even the electrical activity of my brain's neural tissue speeds up. My body responds to the context of the slope and the force of gravity. The movement of my body tells my brain what to do as much as my brain tells my body.

The field of mobile robots has come a long way since 2005. But the shift away from Cartesian mind/body dualism "I think therefore I am" view of intelligence was well underway even then. Exploring the MIT bookstore after the museum visit, I found side by side on the shelf one book called *How the Body Shapes the Mind* (2005) by Shaun Gallagher, a philosophy professor exploring embodiment, and another called *How the Body Shapes the Way We Think: A New View of Intelligence* (2007) by two leading researchers in the field of artificial intelligence. The authors,

Pfeifer and Bongard, argue in favor of embodiment's key role in human and artificial intelligence. They describe embodied intelligence through the interactions between brain, body, and environment:

> [B]ehavior in animals and robots cannot be reduced to internal mechanism alone. Behavior is the result of an agent interacting with the real world, which includes not only the agent's neural system but also its entire body: how the sensors are distributed, the material properties of the muscle-tendon system and the joints and so on. This collection of interdependent mechanisms is referred to as the agent's embodiment. (Pfeiffer & Bongard, 2007, p.75)

Although they use more formal terms than I might, Pfeiffer and Bongard's perspective was similar to what I have been arguing here: the brain is not the whole story. To my surprise, many references in their book were familiar to me. I had not expected such overlap with the papers that Hubert had been sharing for years on coordination, perception, and how movement skills develop. Far from representing either an esoteric or an "alternative" point of view, the perspective about movement that Hubert had been exploring was on the leading edge of mainstream science.

What I discovered was that researchers from many fields were turning away from the "to understand it, break it down" approach. For Rolfers and movement teachers, for the artificial intelligence researchers designing mobile robots, for cognitive scientists and ecological psychologists studying perceptual processes or working in rehabilitation, there was a convergence of interest in the burgeoning field called "dynamic systems." Esther Thelen (1941–2004), one of a group of researchers applying dynamic systems theory to human development, wrote that dynamic systems theories sought "to understand the overall behavior of a system...by asking how and under what circumstances parts cooperate to produce a whole pattern" (Thelen, 1998, p.38). This approach contrasted with traditional ones that broke systems down into parts in order to understand them, which, as we have seen, was often unsuccessful (Thelen, 1998, p.38).

Thelen's work pushed back against the cerebral mystique and included the specific context and environment of the developing child as part of the inquiry into how children grow and learn. Exploring her research in more depth will help us understand something about the dynamic systems perspective and how it might apply to our own movement study. As we will see, the information is compelling enough to inspire growing

partnerships between robotics researchers and those in infant development and cognition.

FISH TANKS AND TREADMILLS: DYNAMIC SYSTEMS THEORY IN ACTION

Our conceptual framework shapes what we do (Thelen, 2005). Like Dr.
Rolf, Thelen was moved to re-examine some of the premises in her field.
One of her experiments investigated a phenomenon called newborn stepping. It had been noted that if you hold a newborn baby upright with
their legs hanging and then let their feet touch the table, you will see the
baby step, as if walking. But after the first few months of life, the stepping
reflex seems to disappear. Traditionally, this observation was explained
as a result of a maturing nervous system. In a classic version of cerebral
mystique, the assumption was that the changes in behavior were due to
the brain's maturation.

To investigate what else might be behind the observation, Thelen created an ingenious experiment using a very large fish tank filled with water.
When she held an older infant—who supposedly had matured beyond the
stepping reflex stage—with their legs hanging in the water, the stepping
reflex showed up again. In another variation, she attached a small weight
to a younger infant's leg—who supposedly still had the reflex—and the
infant no longer showed any stepping motions, as if the reflex had disappeared. What did this mean? In both cases, the parameter that changed
was the weight of the baby's leg—the effect of gravity. The reflex had not
disappeared; rather, it was modified by the context.

Thelen's fish tank experiment disproved the misguided but pervasive
hypothesis that the stepping reflex disappeared due to changes in the brain
alone. Until then, developmental researchers just had not considered that
the weight of the leg—which became greater as the infant grew—was
responsible for the observed change. Development is a complex interaction among a multiplicity of variables. In a different position relative to
gravity, such as being held upright, the baby's growth—the increase in the
weight of the leg—will be a factor. When lying down, the stepping reflex
appears as kicking. Lying down, the movement isn't affected by the baby's
growth. Changing the environment or the situation—taking weight away
in the water or adding a weight or just changing position—will also have
an influence on the baby's behavior.

In their paper celebrating Thelen's work after her death, Spencer and colleagues summarized her important contribution: "Esther [Thelen] ultimately proposed that stepping—like any other behavioral pattern—is not something one has. Rather, *behavior emerges in the moment from the self-organization of multiple components*" (Spencer *et al.*, 2006, p.1523).

Behavior isn't contained inside the baby: it *emerges* as an interaction among many parameters. The initial posture, the muscles and tendons, and the body's weight (i.e., the effect of gravity) combine and recombine in novel ways in different postures and with different movements. Thelen wrote: "in development, everything counts! It is not enough to ascribe change to just the nervous system, because behavior emerges from interactions" (Thelen, 1998, p.37).

In earlier work exploring infant kicking, Thelen had noted how stereotypical the movements seemed, patterns repeating over and over. But when she looked at which muscles were working, to her surprise, she found chaos: flexors and extensors would fire together in seeming opposition, or the baby's leg would extend with no muscles firing at all. How could this be? The patterns of muscle firing were much less systematic than the kicking itself.

Far from the standard idea that a given muscle will fire to produce a consistent movement, as the anatomy books might lead us to believe, in this case, the muscular strategy was variable but the outcome—the kicking—stayed consistent. Thelen wrote: "The traditional view has got it backward, I thought. The body has to instruct the brain" (Thelen, 1998, p.36). Legs behave like levers and springs. Gravity, momentum, and elasticity are moment-to-moment factors that are changing. How could the brain have a plan for everything a baby will encounter? The limbs can't wait for a command from higher up to respond to a situation. Experiencing the situation taught the baby how their body would respond. Thelen realized that the babies had to learn from the situations how their bodies responded. Experiencing the situation was the basis of infants acquiring the skill to grasp objects or sit or walk, and not a genetic program operating independently.

The existing top-down model of human development couldn't account for Thelen's observations, so she turned toward dynamic systems. The basic principles of dynamic systems theory point out that everything is connected and constantly changing, and that small changes can lead to big effects. Dynamic systems self-organize without needing a central controller or command center. Dynamic systems theory provides an alternative approach to the assumption that the brain makes things happen dissociated from any context. Thelen spent a summer studying with J. A. Scott Kelso, an expert on dynamic systems, founder of the Center for Complex Systems and Brain Sciences at Florida Atlantic University, and author of the 1995 book *Dynamic Patterns: The Self-Organization of Brain and Behavior*, to further her understanding of this challenging perspective. The approach of dynamic systems explores how patterns of behavior emerge. Thelen's work with Kelso provided strategies for recognizing the important variables that were functionally relevant to human development.

In other research, Thelen invented a tiny treadmill, just the right size for a baby, that could sit on top of a table. "You can imagine our excitement and delight when the baby who was about 7 months old, and who didn't move a muscle when held upright without the treadmill, responded immediately to the treadmill with beautifully coordinated and alternating steps!" wrote Thelen (1998, p.39). With their feet on the moving platform, babies showed coordination far beyond what was expected for their age. Even with two treadmills side by side moving at different speeds, the babies' legs each adapted to the pace of their own particular ground. The environmental conditions prompted the behavior, not the maturation of the nervous system.

Like Hubert's work showing that people have different strategies for uprightness, Thelen recognized that the specific circumstances and individual differences matter. In a dynamic system, there simply can't be just one right way for every child to develop. This was a dramatic philosophical reframing. She likened a baby's development to jazz improvisation: "as with jazz, the music infants create as they learn to move and explore must be considered as a whole pattern rather than a sequence of individual notes" (Thelen, 1998, p.38). Thelen's work was influential in pushing back against the pre-programmed computer model of development.

Dynamic systems theory was decidedly compelling for Thelen and researchers in many other fields (Edelman, 1992; Goldfield, 1995; Pfeifer & Bongard, 2007; Reed, 1996). Freed from the image in which the executive brain managed all activity, researchers in robotics, neuroscience, rehabilitation, and psychology were inspired by this framework that considered interactions, and in which the situation and initial conditions[3] mattered.

Dynamic systems theory makes a place for embodiment, for understanding that action, perception, and cognition form a whole that cannot be understood by dividing it. Thelen's creative experiments pushed back against accepted explanations of human development and gave confidence to other researchers that it was possible to study whole systems without breaking them into pieces. After years of exposure to objectification and standardization as primary research tools and the only legitimated form of knowing, many scientists as well as movement practitioners like me were given heart by Thelen's work.

Thelen went on to train to become a Feldenkrais practitioner,[4] to apply her work in development to rehabilitation. Sadly, she passed away before she could pursue this passion as well as her expressed interest in using robots to explore how humans learn. Colleagues such as Linda Smith have carried on Thelen's inquiry into the present time.

A DYNAMIC SYSTEMS APPROACH TO EMBODIMENT

The language of dynamic systems applies just as well to our movement as it does to the creation of mobile robots and to infant development. In the context of the MIT class, looking at the issues arising in building mobile systems, and the research base of Gibson and Thelen, helped give substance to alternative ways of imagining movement for the mechanical engineers. What if we consider embodiment itself as a dynamic process, something that emerges from the interaction among many variables? Could it change the way we approach exercising? Could the metaphor of dynamic systems provide a useful framework for somatic practices, to help us consider the relationship among the many variables that go into embodiment and to remind us to include our context as part of movement?

Language such as "perception, action, and cognition" and "sensitivity to initial conditions" helped me to describe my experience of Hubert's approach to movement. When I explored movement work with the stick (see Introduction), for instance, I began from a particular orientation in gravity (standing) and the stick was a parameter, a variable that changed the movement, eliciting new coordinations almost like the treadmill did for the infants in Esther Thelen's study. The initial conditions included the way we touched the stick and the floor—touching and being touched—which could change the whole experience. This is important because it makes space for each one of us: the particular attitude and the specific context we bring to the movement that is occurring impacts the mechanics of the movement. Gravity, the more ubiquitous context, is also a factor. A change in imagining the weight of the stick, floating or heavy, changed the pattern of muscles firing. In the process, the phenomenon we call "core support" *emerged* without any direct, deliberate intention.

Movement occurs as an interaction among these variables. That's what needs to be cultivated: multiple ways of combining and recombining the variables, to practice responding to the moment at hand.

TRY THIS

Go back to the *Stick work* embodiment practice in the Introduction.

Allow yourself to explore this embodiment, noticing your experience.

What would it mean to allow "emergence" as you contact the stick?

What role can the context have in your movement? If you can, go outside! What is it like to include the different context?

What happens when we apply the dynamic systems perspective to staying upright and walking? What are the important parameters we will discover that organize this complex movement? That's the topic of the next chapter, in which we will turn to robotics again.

CHAPTER TWO

Body in Gravity

How do we keep our balance in gravity? Stabilizing ourselves or managing our instability is a key feature of our biped mobile system. As Hubert put it, "The problem for a biped in gravity isn't how to stand up, it's how not to fall down." Hubert's elegant statement hides the serious nature of falls: they are a leading cause of death for humans around the world (World Health Organization, 2021). For all organisms living on the face of this planet, not falling down is the prime directive for movement, but it's easier on four or more legs than it is on two. As long as it's working, we don't really notice balancing as an essential aspect of every other movement. It just happens.

In this chapter, we are going to use biped robots for movement analysis in order to reveal what goes on below the level of consciousness for us humans as we navigate our environment. We will go on to explore the research basis that shows how the very same pathways that we use to organize our uprightness also serve as our first expression and communication channels, in contrast to our robot friends. Following Hubert, we call this complexity of human experience—relating to gravity's information and relating to each other—tonic function.

HOW NOT TO FALL DOWN

For a moving body in a gravitational field, the problem is not having good posture or how to stay straight, but *how not to fall down.* The experience of gravity is not alignment; it is keeping our balance. Balancing is not static—find it and keep it—but dynamic, an ongoing activity.

Standing and breathing are a balancing act, an interaction with gravity that we are engaged in, consciously or not. Balancing is not "holding a center," but finding and leaving, constantly discovering a dynamic combination of variables that works for the moment.

TRY THIS

Stand up and experience this for yourself.

Take a moment to notice. Can you feel the floor under your feet?

Where is your weight—more on your toes or your heels? More on the outside of your feet or the inside? Is there more weight on one foot or the other, or is your weight evenly distributed?

Are your knees locked? What happens if you allow some ease in your knees?

Are you keeping yourself still? Scan through your body. Is there any holding that you can let go of? Let yourself sigh, all the way down to your ankles.

With the next breath, you may find yourself swaying. How are you moving through the breath cycle: exhaling; pausing; inhaling and exhaling again?

Give yourself time for a few breaths. Find out if you can feel the balancing act as your weight shifts through the changing sensations in the soles of your feet as they touch the floor.

For contrast, deliberately hold yourself still. Does the added tension change the breath?

BIPED ROBOTS

After my teaching experience at MIT, I continued to follow robotics and specifically the development of humanoid mobile robots with great fascination. In 2016, invited to present on the topic of "Shaping Perception" for an interdisciplinary seminar for the Kahn Liberal Arts Institute at Smith College, I again turned to robots. Bipeds are an unusual phenomenon in the animal world—we don't really have another animal to compare ourselves with in order to get insight into how much is involved in navigating our environment on two legs. Looking at the history of humanoid robot design brings hidden dimensions of embodiment to light.

A biped robot has a different set of problems from the Roboroach and robotic tuna. The tuna lives and moves in a watery environment with very different physics compared to our terrestrial one. The cockroach uses six legs to manage its terrestrial environment. Staying up, for bipeds like us, is not easy! Navigating on two legs is harder than it looks—and more interesting. For a person, staying upright is a mechanical challenge, but as we shall see, also much more.

A big challenge for the early designers of humanoid biped robots was how to make a robot that didn't fall over. Maintaining balance on two legs is so difficult that many robotics companies gave up on creating bipedal machines altogether, and instead use quadrupeds or completely different styles of locomotion, such as wheels. But some companies have persisted and continue to appreciate all that goes into yours and my everyday movements, while the rest of us take it all for granted.

While preparing the Kahn Institute talk back in 2016, I came across a video compilation of numerous biped robot falls from the first day of the 2015 Defense Advanced Research Projects Agency (DARPA) Challenge, a robotics competition (IEEE Spectrum, 2015). The Challenge came about after the 2011 Fukushima nuclear power plant meltdown following a terrible tsunami in Japan. U.S. Department of Defense specialists wondered if it would have been possible to change the course of events if there had been a robot capable of assisting the first responders.

The YouTube video, set to lively piano music and dubbed "hilarious" by the press, quickly went viral. There's something about watching the robots fall that has an odd appeal. They look like us, but there are important differences. Apart from its comedic value, the video offers a wonderful chance for movement analysis: what is missing in the robots' movements jumps out and reveals the underpinnings of our own movements. I was curious enough to seek out the recording of the whole event to find examples of the robots in motion (and how they failed) to show at my talk. I was in luck (DARPAtv, 2015).

DARPA had put up $3.5 million in prize money to promote development of a robot with the necessary capabilities to respond to an emergency like the one at Fukushima. The robots were given seven tasks, including to drive and get out of a buggy, turn a valve, cut a hole in a wall, walk over rubble, and climb a flight of stairs. The 2015 competition was the culmination of a multi-year project, the result of a huge effort over four years, with 25 teams and hundreds of contributing engineers, scientists, and volunteers.

In all the early competitions, the robots were tethered, but in the finals, they had to complete their tasks with no safety line. Some robots eventually completed the tasks, but it turned out to be harder than the teams expected: a lot of robots fell down.

Car trouble

In the YouTube video, a cheer goes up from the crowd in the bleachers as a red jeep inches across the black-and-white checkered finish line. It's a clear June day in Pomona, California. Color-coded competition courses are set up like a track-and-field event around the fairground. On the red course, the robot driver slides over to the jeep's doorway, begins to stand up very slowly, arms in the air, then lurches out of the vehicle and falls face first on the hard-packed dirt, twitching uncontrollably. Meet Running Man, the robot from team IHMC-USA, one of the winners of the competition.

What's so hard about getting out of a car? Many of us do it daily without thinking. But the engineers reported that getting out of the buggy was one of the hardest tasks for the robots. It requires balance and coordination, and subtle weight shifts that are among the hardest to control. The micro-movements involved in keeping its balance while sliding on the seat toward the door require the robot's computer controller to send a multitude of messages: shift right, shift left, then right, et cetera. With all the weight shifts involved and then standing up, the computer can't cope. The robot shakes and falls over.

> **TRY THIS**
> Now compare your experience: count the number of weight shifts involved as you get out of your chair. As you sit down again, notice how much control you use as you return to your chair. At what point do you "fall" into the chair? Standing up and sitting down are a complex coordination.

Be glad that things were a little easier for you when you learned how not to fall down! Just like Robotuna and Roboroach, Running Man shows us what we don't usually appreciate about ourselves. Why don't we fall down more? Why are these tasks easy for us but complicated for a robot?

CENTER OF GRAVITY

In another video segment of the competition, Running Man takes on the stair challenge. The IHMC robot is humanoid, with two legs and two arms that end in a kind of gripper. It has a black torso and metallic limbs and appears to be carrying a large white backpack—its power supply—connected with many tubes and wires. Just lifting its foot to climb the first step sends it sprawling over onto its back, tipped over by the change in its center of gravity.

Our center of gravity is one of the most basic elements of balancing that we humans have a sense for in movement but that is mostly missing in the robots. An object's center of gravity is an imaginary point at which weight is evenly spread out, keeping the object in balance.[1] Another way to see center of gravity is in relation to the base of support, a variable that will change depending on what we are doing. Our sense for balance is so subtle and sophisticated that it is mostly able to manage all the changes induced by our own limbs, by our plan of action, and by different environmental factors like wind without much conscious attention. Thanks to millions of years of evolution, our systems know what information to pay attention to and how to interpret it—very quickly! Most of us spent our early years honing this inheritance into a personal skill.

How do we do it? As we approach a stair, a complex anticipatory process is already taking place. We predict from experience what changes will be needed: by the time our leg is lifting, our torso is already compensating to manage the anticipated shift in balance. For the robot to climb a stair, its programming lifts its leg from the hip. For us, following our gaze and intention to act, spine and trunk would already be involved without our voluntary direction. (Though humanoid, the robot doesn't have a spine per se.) A human being, even a young one, has had hours of practice learning a preparatory gesture that anticipates a change in balance.

Watching the robot, I perceive the missing movement through its absence: through my own expectation/anticipation/feeling of the motion of a person climbing the stairs, I can tell this robot is going to fail at the instant the foot comes up, almost before it falls backwards. This is part of what makes the fall funny: I already know what is going to happen through my own body's response. Watching other bodies is an additional source of information for us about our own bodies, from very early infancy. We feel in ourselves what we see in others. In 2015, Running Man did not have this benefit. Feeling our gravity center, anticipating and compensating for changes in our balance, is part of our daily movement that most of us take for granted. The clumsiness of early robot design makes visible this complex set of processes that usually goes on for us without a second thought as we move around in the world.

PRE-MOVEMENT, PREPARING FOR ACTION

In the 1980s, V. S. Gurfinkel published research describing our capacity to predict the effect of a movement on our center of gravity. He called it "anticipatory postural activity" and carefully measured it with electromyography (Gurfinkel, 1994). For instance, standing at the fridge, reaching for the milk to pour in your coffee cup, the first muscles to contract are not the ones that move your arm, but muscles in your legs and trunk that manage the shift in center of gravity engendered by the change in your arm position—and these muscles engage even before you begin to lift your arm. Not falling over has to be managed first. The anticipation precedes the intended action. Hubert called this crucial and ongoing process *pre-movement*. Every moment and every movement must include the need to not fall over.

Our system is constantly anticipating and predicting how our movement will change our balance, but ordinarily, we don't give it much thought. In the robot, this preparation was obviously missing. Yet this management of our center of gravity goes on all day, for better or worse, in each of us. It's not quite a "reflex" because it is learned, not hardwired. Not falling over conceals our ongoing conversation with gravity, an active process we are engaged in below the level of consciousness. Unlike heartbeat and digestion, which go on even in our sleep, managing our uprightness is a process we are actively participating in at this very moment, even as I write and you read this material.

Even though the complex process of keeping our balance comes naturally, that doesn't mean we are doing it that well, even when we are just walking. Human movement that could be effortless is often accomplished with a lot of unnecessary effort. But the importance of pre-movement, an ongoing relationship with gravity in humans, is revealed by the robots' failure! Most of the time, we behave as if that whole dimension of life does not even exist. Yet in practice, to change any of our patterns—physical, emotional, or otherwise—the pre-movements are exactly what needs our attention. Once an action is underway, the process is harder to influence.

TRY THIS ✓

To experience your own pre-movements, stand behind the back of your chair or in front of your desk or table with your palms lightly in contact with the object.

Now, imagine that you are going to push this object across your room.

With this intention and before you even begin to move, pause and notice the subtle bodily shifts, tensions, or sensations this imagined task brings, as you anticipate the action and effort involved.

That's your way of preparing to push—your pre-movement—and it includes not falling down.

PROBLEMS IN PERCEPTION

On the yellow track, Japan's Team NEDO-JSK robot, Jaxon, approaches the valve-turning task. Jaxon is the same humanoid design as Running Man, only with purple detailing on the arms and head. We see a robot, up on two legs that are bent where our knees would be, move toward a red valve shaped like a wheel. How incredibly slow it is. The robot pauses for a long time, preparing. Then it takes several steps in relatively quick succession, and there is another long pause. The head component tilts and its camera whirls.

The grippers prepare and the robot moves forward with very small steps, just to the left of the valve. The robot arm carefully reaches for the valve, only it misses. The robot has moved just a little too far to the left and there has been no self-correction. We see the robot's head jerk down, and its eyes (the camera) fixate on the valve. As it goes to turn the valve, it misses the wheel entirely. Still about a foot to the left of it, the robot goes through the motions of turning the valve in the air anyway. It begins the slow movements to turn the wheel that isn't there, and within a second the momentum of its arms turning counterclockwise topples it right over. It slowly crashes down, the turn continuing into a pathetic partial cartwheel of its very expensive frame.

What were the engineers thinking? How did Jaxon miss the valve? How could it be that its sensors didn't detect that it was not in touch with the object it was meant to be turning? Any toddler would certainly notice that they had missed the wheel: seeing and reaching, perception and action, come together with the need to maintain our uprightness in human development. Perception and action are linked: at only a few months old, a baby only reaches for objects within the space of its grasp (von Hofsten, 1979, cited in Reed, 1982). So why doesn't the robot do what even toddlers do: plan ahead to compensate for the force of the turn? An older child would automatically create some stability as they turned the wheel, subconsciously activating different muscle groups or leaning in the opposite direction of the turn to manage the anticipated forces. The engineers missed all these key elements of movement. Watching the robots, the missing connections between planning actions, perceiving the environment, and anticipating the effects of gravity are suddenly very easy to see.

PERCEPTION AND EMOTION

Not least, once the fall begins, these robots make no attempt to stop it. The robots do not resist a fall or try to right themselves at the moment the fall begins. It's as if they surrender to fate. There's no pumping of arms, no startle reflex or preparatory organization that would be seen in a person, who would know, through sensations before thinking, that balance was in jeopardy.

If we trip on the sidewalk, a series of emergency maneuvers immediately ensues in an attempt to keep us upright. Depending on the direction of our momentum, our inner ear and receptors in the soles of our feet signal our trunk muscles, front or back, to quickly tense, counteracting the momentum and hopefully avoiding the anticipated fall. And if we sensed failure in these uprighting maneuvers, in a fraction of an instant, our arms might stretch out to break the fall. In 2015, none of this was part of the robots' programming.

For us, not falling over is more than just a mechanical exercise. If I trip, there is a feeling of fear—uh-oh!—even before thinking begins. Keeping our balance in gravity is tied up with our emotional arousal system: the feeling of falling is a feeling of being out of control. It generally triggers a sense of alarm, an autonomic reaction, and an immediate righting response. Perception and emotion come together. If we have learned how to respond to these signals, it can become a source of fun, whether snowboarding or riding a bike. It all depends on how we relate to the signals that help us not fall down.

The robots in the video did not "know" they were falling or have any feelings about it. Maybe that's also part of what made them fun to watch. As they fall, there is no one there reacting to the sense of losing balance; no one there anticipating being hurt; no one there feeling embarrassed, imagining people watching and laughing at their clumsiness.

The failure of these early bipedal robots reveals that there is a whole dimension underlying movement that the engineers missed. And they're not alone: unless something is going wrong, we don't tend to notice how much is happening beneath the surface. We take balancing (i.e., working with gravity) and perception for granted, and in 2015 these qualities were not yet part of the robots' design. However, the robots' failures remind us of their significance: their falls bring into focus how much perceiving the environment shapes our own movements in ways that are hidden in plain sight.

The DARPA competition tasks presented the researchers with a series of mechanical problems: the robots had to contend with controlling degrees of freedom, perceiving and navigating the landscape, and manipulating objects, all without falling over. For a human being, embodiment includes all these things—sensing gravity, balancing, perceiving and responding to the environment. But it doesn't start with mechanics. For us, it starts with moving and responding to the environment as far back as the womb. Once we are born, the signals change dramatically: we go from pressure everywhere to the unidirectional pull of gravity (H. Godard, workshop November 1993). That pull becomes information that we use as we learn to orient our eyes, hands, and trunk for action in the world.

TONIC FUNCTION: GRAVITY, EXPRESSION, CONNECTION

In a human being, perception and action and gravity's signals are all nested together. They are also entwined with emotions on the simplest level and part of our connection with other people. For example, a baby kicks faster to express excitement, using the same kicking movements Esther Thelen examined in her research (Chapter One). The very same system the baby will eventually use to stand up is part of an expressive system. The baby's caretakers may match or miss these early expressions, shaping the child's experience of other people.

All these dimensions factor into what we call "body" when we see each other. Watching another human being, we see the physical management of balance as posture, and that posture reflects a history, habitual attitudes, the way we meet the world. Staying upright goes far beyond the mechanical phenomenon of not falling over. It is part of what shapes our sense of self, an essential element of the whole human project.

Hubert adopted "tonic function" as a shorthand label for his broad perspective. Reflex muscle contraction—muscle tone or tonic postural activity[2]—is part of what allows us to maintain our uprightness, along with many other elements of our physiology. The cerebellum, basal ganglia, thalamus, and the tonic muscles that are full of muscle spindles sensitive to the stretch reflex all participate in our ability to stay upright. Many areas of peripheral and central nervous system, bone, ligament, and muscle combine into a system that manages our ability to stay upright in changing circumstances—the tonic system. What was different in Hubert's perspective was bringing in the expressive aspect of this very same postural system.

The term tonic function was originally coined by French developmental psychologist Henri Wallon (1879–1962). Wallon observed that during our first months of life, the small variations in muscle tone[3] that later help us stand up are not in service of intentional actions such as reaching for a cup. The subtle movements of changing tone are our earliest form of expression, our first communication channels with the people on whom we depend. Imagine a parent picking up an infant from a crib. As they gently slip their hands under the baby's body, the infant responds by adjusting muscle tone—perhaps stiffening slightly, then relaxing into the parent's arms. The parent, sensing the baby's initial tension, shifts their hold, cradling the infant more securely. In turn, the baby's muscles relax further, settling in comfortably against the caregiver (Wallon, 1956).

De Ajuriaguerra (1911–1993), a Spanish-French neuropsychiatrist, called this exchange—the back-and-forth adjustment through which the caregiver and baby continuously "tune in" to each other's tension and relaxation through changing qualities of muscle tone—a dialogue, a "tonic dialogue." Neither speaks a word, yet a meaningful exchange takes place through the language of posture, touch, and tone.

Like Wallon and De Ajuriaguerra, André Bullinger (1941–2015) was a pioneering Swiss neuropsychologist and developmental theorist whose work significantly contributed to our understanding of early childhood development, particularly in the areas of sensorimotor integration and embodiment. In the perspective described in his collected essays (2010), Bullinger described how even before birth, from the very beginning in the womb's watery environment, every variation in the sensory flow, whether from inside or outside, causes an increase in tone in the developing organism. The fetus already responds to changes in the environment through withdrawal or approach, moving away or towards. For example, in response to irritants, one postural reflex causes extension in the back muscles. Interestingly, in utero this extension causes the fetus to encounter the wall of the uterus in a kind of meeting, the very first tonic dialogue. By the time a baby is born, she already has a repertory of reflexes, ways of responding, and postures such as extension that have been practiced.

The repertory of postures I have described are based in reflex: they happen of themselves, without intention. The work of the first year of a baby's life is to build on that repertory: to use the support the human environment provides and the innate talents with which each baby comes into the world to begin to make sense of and take action in that environment. The function of "tone," a key element in our ability to keep our balance in motion, includes a complex human experience that connects a baby with her surroundings and caretakers, and is the first communication channel. From the very beginning of life, the body is responsive and expressive.

A baby communicating with adults through subtle changes in tone is a very different image of the body from that of mobile robots! Like the toddler in Van Gogh's painting (see Introduction), many of us have made the journey from a babe in arms to an autonomous upright individual, from a human embrace to the embrace of the field of gravity.

The neuropsychiatrist and psychoanalyst Judith Kestenberg's (1910–1999) research also explored the infant's experience. Over years of interacting with babies and watching parents and infants move together, Kestenberg described links between the movements of the physical body, emotional expression, and psychological development. The baby's moving toward something or shrinking away from it is an expressive process. Bound flow—when opposing muscle pairs of agonist and antagonist contract simultaneously—contrasted with free flow. Both capacities are needed in everyday movements—for example, to pick up an object—but the two qualities of flow are also a means of expression: flinging our arms wide in a free-flow welcome, or the careful control of bound flow to learn to shape letters. Kestenberg connected her observations of infants to the movements of the adults she worked with. The resulting psycho-logical profile based on movement patterns, the Kestenberg Movement Profile, can describe an adult as well as an infant. For each one of us, the shaping of our body's tone—our use of tonic movements—begins in our first movements as an infant. These become familiar pathways that stay with us as we grow up, shaping our gestural style and our repertory of possible actions.

Interpreting this research and working with Hubert brought home to me that we simply cannot work on the tonic system from a purely mechanical point of view. Our humanness, our way of perceiving the world, and our sense of ourselves are intimately tied up with the system we use for staying upright and in motion. Although comparing ourselves with robots reveals aspects of movement we take for granted, to be human is something else. We evolved as humans on this planet, organized at the deepest level to use gravity's signals for perception and in service of movement and relationship. As we will see, in our dynamic embodiment, managing gravity's pull, perceiving, preparing for action, and being in relationship with other people and our surroundings are all important variables that we can work with in the service of expanding our move-ment repertory.

EMBODIMENT: PUSHING THE CHAIR

Years ago, the embodiment practice described below brought home to me the many dimensions of center of gravity in a person's experience.

Another day, another classroom, this time in Philadelphia, in 1993. Hubert took a metal folding chair and invited us to push it around the room. Such a simple idea, like pushing a cart at the supermarket. But there was so much to it! The instruction "push a heavy object" evoked enormous effort in our bodies before we even touched the chair. We felt the anticipation that launched us into tension: anticipating the amount of force that would be involved—which happened involuntarily—led to a tightening of the front of the body, a curling toward the chair along with the tension and preparation in the upper surface of hands and wrists. The chair was awkward; the floor resisted the movement.

Like the practice with the stick, Hubert then suggested we let the feel-ing of the chair come into our hands, while staying with our own center of gravity. Instead of leaning forward onto the chair back, trying to get the chair to move, we stayed over our own two feet, keeping the sense of the space behind us while accepting the cold metal into our hands. All of a sudden, the chair moved across the floor almost effortlessly. (This is a great practice for the supermarket with an actual shopping cart.)

Hubert explained that when we lean on the chair with tension, we inadvertently end up with one center of gravity between two separate entities. "You are trying to share a center of gravity," he said. He called that fusion.

We can use different sources of information to keep our balance, but some of them will work better than others. There may be unintended consequences in very simple actions. As we saw earlier in this chapter, our physical experiences can carry an emotional message. Having someone to lean on, for example. But what if who or what we are leaning on moves? Imagine if our sense of such a basic security—how not to fall down—depends directly on another person! Every time they move, we would have to move to keep our balance. This could be very stressful!

The alternative is to stay centered over our own feet and in touch with the ground, while at the same time making receptive contact with the chair the way we practiced with the stick of wood. This sequence allowed us to keep our own center of gravity while affecting the other (the chair, in this case).

For Rolfers who do hands-on work, the exercise had layers of application far beyond the chair. In daily practice with our clients, we use a variety of touch: sometimes our hands are receiving and taking in information, sometimes we are exerting pressure, and at all times we need to find our own center and make space for the client's experience. Being in relationship while keeping our own center is significant for both our work and our personal lives.

Articulation

Another word for joint—where two bones meet and allow movement—is articulation. And to function, an articulation requires a separation. Many years ago, in a tango lesson with expert teacher Daniel Trenner, he told me that my job was to help my partner have the best possible posture. Instead of leaning on my partner, I was to stay with my own base of support. The strength arising from finding my own footing would translate to my partner. It was a very different interpretation of leading and following in dance. As a follower, I had an important contribution to make. By staying with my own center of gravity, I was actually helping the leader do their job.

TRY THIS   ✓

If you have a chair or something that rolls or can slide on the floor, use that. If not, stand behind the back of your chair or in front of your desk or table with your palms lightly in contact with the object.

Before you begin to push, bring your awareness to the ground meeting the soles of your feet. Sense the space all around you—the light, the sounds, the air moving. As you lightly make contact with the object, pause to receive it—feel it touching you.

With this preparation, imagine or begin to allow the object to move across the room. Notice if the preparation for the action results in a different felt sense throughout your body than what you experienced from the exploration earlier in this chapter.

If you are using a chair or object that can slide, notice if you can feel the difference between sharing a center of gravity and keeping your own while you push the chair.

Recalling the image from the Van Gogh painting, a relationship requires a separation. Supported by the mother, the child shares one center of gravity. Leaving the mother's support, she must meet the challenges of managing uprightness, her own relationship to gravity's signals. She can't come into her own relationship with gravity until she leaves the security of the shared center. Yet the painting depicts where she is going—not too far! The key is being in relationship while maintaining your own center of gravity.

Upright

In spite of their awkwardness, we recognize the human figure in the robots described in this chapter, yet the image of a robot only serves to emphasize the differences with a human being (Cross *et al.*, 2011). Contrast the image of a machine, however endearing, with the image of a six-month-old infant. Mechanics alone cannot capture an infant's alive curiosity and discovery of their surroundings. Human animals are embedded in their relationships and in the terrestrial environment. Our curriculum after birth is to learn to use gravity's provocative signals as a foil, first to lift our heads and eventually to maintain our balance—the signals teach us where we are by threatening imbalance. Not falling down and staying in touch with our environment through perception and action are our inheritance. A baby is not a blank slate but an actively selecting animate being. Growing up is learning to use the information the environment provides while performing ever more complex actions—from just sitting up while grasping objects to walking and running without falling and then on to bicycle riding and speaking and so on, with managing our instability always part of every action. Human relations throughout the lifespan likewise require a balancing act between autonomy and relatedness that is both metaphorical and physical.

CHAPTER THREE

Managing Instability

So how do we stay upright while in motion? Before you read any further, try to answer in your own words: What keeps us upright?

For the most part, walking just happens, unless something goes wrong. Once it is learned, we don't have to think about it. Walking becomes a steady presence, a capacity akin to heartbeat, blood flow, digestion. Babies practice—but without thinking in words about it. Walking ability marks a huge change for each child: it's the first moment of independence, as crawling and toddling allow exploring a larger terrain, and, as any parent knows, when baby-proofing stairs and outlets and cabinets becomes unavoidable! For a human being, the mechanics of walking are associated with other people. Getting up on our own two feet is a symbolic event, as we saw in Van Gogh's painting "First Steps." None of this is present for the robots, but when we watch them, we almost imbue the mechanical systems with the same triumph we ourselves experienced in getting upright.

As adults now, even though we walk without thinking of it, a lot still goes on beneath the surface. This chapter unpacks the important subconscious dimensions of walking, taking an experiential point of view and an evolutionary perspective, as well as exploring how perception and balance enter into every step—all of which was missing from the robots. We will discover that the very way we see is intimately connected with navigating our environment and with our emotional response as we move through the world.

TAKING A WALK

When I am walking, certain sensations float into my awareness, and certain words and images guide me: the miraculous sensations of the heel finding its lengthening into the ground and the toes finding their line, the one that lets them stretch out or forward. How that, in and of itself, brings the transfer of weight to the other foot. A remarkable feeling, because it is the feeling of walking that happens, not walking of my doing. Waiting for the heels to be lengthened: the heels make contact, and keep going, as if following a line drawn through the earth itself. Then walking begins, the forefoot, the propeller—and the rest follows automatically—forward momentum, but not "teetering on the edge of catastrophe" (Napier, 1967, p.55), because that heel is still reaching to the center of the earth. All that's left for me to do is to start again and again to find the way it goes. The lightest of intentions—heel and ground—and the movement is there. With this attunement, something else comes to me...

The Arnold Arboretum, where I like to go walking, is a feast in springtime. The trees call from every direction as I walk: buds, blooms, splashes of color, yellow, or wafting lilac scent. Spring comes upon me full of sensory delights.

I like the feeling, especially the second moment—the one after my attention has been grabbed. Then I might pause, breathe in, or go closer, drawn to put my nose right into a buxom blossom. Or I stop and look, but it is not so much looking—not peering—as waiting...and in a little while, like a lens focusing, something else appears, beyond the initial attraction. Details. The intricate color design at the heart of the tree peony; the particular shade of green and the softness of new leaves of the dawn redwood, masquerading as flat needles, but really leaf-like, not tough at all. In other seasons, what is seen-felt-touched might be the pattern of bare branching, magnificent sculptures, the buds, fuzzy or naked, waiting—or catkins hanging, startling advertisements. This is the world, walking.

BORN TO WALK

Our bodies are made for walking.[1] With each step, the movement of the bones of feet, legs, and spine, honed over hundreds of thousands of years, work with our elastic tissue, which extends, storing kinetic energy that transforms into the next step, each step. The structures of our feet, spine, and arms also have evolved specifically with our upright stance and our nervous system (Tobias, 1982). Hardwired neural programs of rhythm that alternate our arm and leg movements have been working since our time in the womb. Their innate pattern combines with moment-by-moment feedback from and adjustment to the surrounding world. We are a per-petual motion animal, walking nearly for free, evolved to be able to work with gravity.

Our bodies are unstable by design: smaller at the base than at the top. For humans, being upright while moving is a continuous process of letting go. Walking is a balancing act—an artfully managed instability. Although this instability complicates things, it also has a positive side: our essential instability makes walking inherently economical. Instead of lifting each leg against the force of gravity, walking can be elegant falling and quick recovery (Berthoz, 2009/2012).

That is what makes walking an efficient movement and, evolution-arily, a well-adapted one: it doesn't take a lot of energy for us to go from standing to moving. In fact, it's standing still that takes muscular effort to prevent a fall. So falling, or controlled instability, is in a way part of our normal motion as human beings (Gracovetsky, 2007). Grace is revealed in the delicate balance between letting go and control. Have you ever seen a novice on rollerblades? They tense every muscle that isn't engaged in shuffling their feet. Years later, the expert rollerblader seems almost to fly down the street, arms swinging in coordination with the glide of the skates. There's almost no effort or holding at all.

Walking is not driven solely top-down by the brain. Consciously, we set our direction, our intention to go here or there. Fortunately, we don't need to control each of our limbs individually in order to walk. In fact, we can't: if you add up all the joints involved, the total number of individual commands would be too great for the brain to tell each component what to do one at a time. Reflexively, our body's weight, in contact with the ground through our feet, activates special nerve receptors in the soles of our feet that are sensitive to pressure. The pressure receptors signal the muscles in the back and front of the trunk, coordinating falling and recovering. When our feet touch the ground, walking is enabled by the contact—where we meet the world (Thelen & Smith, 1995).

MOVING AND PERCEIVING

If you look with the mind of a scientist, you will see that beyond the shape of us, our very brain and nervous system are also the result of our rela-tionship with this world. Although perceiving and moving may seem like separate activities, scientists tell us that moving is actually the very basis of our capacity to perceive. This is, for instance, what the valve-turning robot Jaxon was missing: in its programming, there was no automatic connection between seeing the valve, grasping it, and the turning action. We take it all for granted until the robot, built without these connections, fails.

Moving may be the evolutionary reason creatures have a brain. For all living creatures, perception depends on the need to make our way in the world: how we go towards and how we go away, how we get from here to there. These are the activities upon which survival depends, and which shape the perceptual systems of living beings in response to their environments.[2] For instance, neuroscientist Rodolfo Llinás tells the story of the sea squirt: this small ocean creature starts out as a larva and goes on to develop into a tadpole with a primitive brain. As it matures, it finds a place to land, to plant itself, and once planted, it digests its brain. Once it stops moving around, it doesn't need a brain. The sea squirt's development suggests that our brains and nervous systems, our organs of perception, evolved specifically as tools to help us navigate our environment (Llinás, 2002).

Our bodies evolved in a terrestrial environment. Being upright on two feet, able to look around and see far off, has been of enormous benefit to our species. This is true at an evolutionary level, and it is also true for each of us in our own development: self-generated movement shapes the development of perception itself.

Perceptual scientists Held and Hein (1963) showed the importance of self-generated movement to proper visual development in a landmark experiment. Pairs of newborn kittens both received the same visual stimulation, but one of the pair explored on their own while the other one was moved about passively in a sling. The passive kittens never learned to see correctly: they could not use vision to guide their paws or detect a cliff. Even their capacity to blink was negatively affected by their lack of active movement.

What is true for kittens is true for babies: humans learn to see through exploring our environment on our own power. As we move through the landscape, our system picks up the structural, invariant patterns of flow, the regular patterns of light and dark: the sky and horizon that orient us but always remain out of reach, and the ground that is present, consistent, patient, like the receptive earth of the I Ching (Wilhelm, 1967, p.307). We use these perceptual cues unconsciously to organize orientation, to know which way is up and which way is down. The sensory/perceptual experience of self-in-motion—the pattern of changes in the environment that become associated with it—allows us to make sense of the world (Reed, 1996).

But the robot's failure shows us that the perception–motion connection was not how the engineers imagined movement. It was not part of their image of the moving body. Traditionally, anatomists distinguished between a central and peripheral nervous system: the central nervous system (CNS) was supposed to integrate the sensory input from the body and send out motor commands for movement. The peripheral nervous system (PNS) was described as conveying sensory information from the body to the CNS. The engineers inherited this reductionist perspective that separated sensory and motor, but when they tried to put it into practice in their robot designs, it failed to produce effective movement. James Gibson and ecological psychologists who followed his perspective would not have been surprised at all. They would emphasize that these distinctions, while useful for understanding the biological underpinnings of perception and action, do not fully capture the holistic nature of our interaction with our environment. Instead, ecological psychology proposes we think in terms of perception and action systems, based on the Russian neurophysiologist Nikolai Bernstein's physiology of activity (instead of passive reactivity) (Reed, 1982). We use our perceptual systems to evaluate and explore, and our action systems to adjust our movements. Unlike a machine that can be turned off, an organism or a human being is always managing a kind of disequilibrium in relation to the environment that requires us to adjust and adapt to ever-changing conditions. In this model, the most fundamental action system is the basic orienting system—because not falling down is key to nearly all our perceptions and actions. That's where our vestibular system helps us out.

Vestibular system

Managing our instability requires more than reflexes, the right-shaped bones, and elastic material. It also depends on a sophisticated perceptual system. The brain's job is not so much to direct the body as it is to pick up the right cues from the environment (Kelso, 1982). Below the level of consciousness, we tune in to information that tells us which way is up. We come equipped with a precision navigational device, the vestibular system, the labyrinth of the inner ear, which combines a linear acceleration monitor and a gyroscope to detect rotation. Three semicircular canals in the inner ear detect motion in three dimensions. One canal picks up on forward and backward motion, one perceives motion on the horizontal plane, and the third picks up movement in the vertical. Little crystals in the inner ear, the otoliths, move in response to gravity. Without our knowing, their weight and movement signal us via hair cells in a fluid medium, keeping our heads stable as our senses take in the world.

Where and What

When we take the perspective of Gibson and ask the question "How do we navigate our environment?" we discover that the receptors and neural pathways involved make up a special system. Ungerleider and Mishkin (1982) confirmed the discovery of two cortical visual systems in primates that have come to be known as Where and What pathways. The Where pathway allows us to perceive the shape and general location of objects. It also registers and responds to movement, but it doesn't link to language. The other pathway, the What system, allows us to recognize and name. It captures the details, the textures and colors, and allows us to identify the objects seen.

This functional distinction helped make sense of what Weiskrantz (1989) called "blindsight" (see Introduction). Although blindsight patients' eyes are undamaged, they cannot see, and yet, paradoxically, they avoid obstacles and orient appropriately to their surroundings. Blindsighted people have lost the function of the What pathway, the one that sees and names, but their Where system continues to guide them in walking and other activities of spatial localization. Since the two functions generally happen together, it has only been through unusual cases such as the blindsighted patients that researchers have understood that the functions of knowing what something is and being able to name it and the ability to take action in relation to something are neurologically separated. The Where and What distinction holds true for the sense of touch and for the other senses (Paillard, 1999, 2005).

For most of us, these two systems operate seamlessly in tandem most of the time. The Where system manages some aspects of navigation for us. It operates with high speed and is thought to be evolutionarily older. Interestingly, that aspect of vision is closely tied with the inner ear's function of maintaining our balance and is linked to peripheral vision. The Where system lets something unforeseen catch our eye. Walking with the Where system, with peripheral vision, we have a wide gaze. We are encountering the world, open to impressions from our landscape. We are available to see something new. The What system then contributes details, precision.

Weapon focus

Usually, Where/peripheral and What/focal vision function comfortably together: peripheral vision gives the context, the wider field, while focal vision detects all the details of a particular object. When playing tennis, for example, peripheral vision is predominant when we go to the net because it allows a faster response, whereas at the baseline we depend more on focal vision because of its precision. But sometimes the smooth working of the systems can get stuck, with consequences to our emotional state.

For example, Schmitz *et al.* (2009) found a correlation between our emotional state and the visual field. Namely, a negative mood was associated with a narrower field of vision. Likewise, in a situation of more extreme danger such as if threatened with a gun, the gun would likely get our full visual, focal attention, while the details of the surroundings would in a sense disappear. In this threatening situation, our focus narrows and peripheral impressions are inhibited. This narrowed view is tellingly called "weapon focus" (Ross *et al.*, 1994).

After a trauma, the visual system does not automatically reset. Instead, we can end up inadvertently stuck with a physiological inhibition of the periphery. The danger message to our autonomic nervous system will shape how we use our eyes. Trauma aside, we may over-focus and shut out the periphery in our daily life with phones and screens. We may come to depend on focal vision too much. If the What system habitually works first or too soon, it can actually inhibit peripheral vision, interfering with the function of the vestibular system, which may lead to further difficulty organizing our stability in motion.

Walking through the world with our eyes anchored this way can have negative repercussions. It may not matter if your eyes are looking at a dangerous weapon or your phone. The narrowing of gaze, losing peripheral vision, may take its toll on us through tension, effort, and fear. We need Where and What gazes to function smoothly together, like a camera moving between zoom function and wide angle. Given the importance of this capacity, it is surprising that for most of us it isn't an ability we think to exercise. Walking can give us an opportunity. Instead of over-emphasizing the eyes' focal use in balance, we can tune in to peripheral vision and other sensory systems: the feeling of the ground and the inner ear.

SURRENDERING TO WALKING

Walking seems so simple, yet it links us to the whole history of our ancestors on this planet and the evolution of our nervous systems. It can bring us back to being deeply in touch with our surroundings. This capacity goes beyond physiology. For the Where system, body and world are not separate, and that which is perceived is self-in-environment, together. This is the place before words, in which there is not a fixed identity, an "I," apart. As Alan Watts wrote, "Your body knows that you are one with the universe" (n.d.). Wide focus, the Where system, keeps us in touch with the world. Well-organized walking allows us to move through the world with the Where brain orienting us, while still able to be drawn to the beauty of the particular through our focal vision.[3]

Andante, lulled by the rhythm of walking, we are engaged in exploration. Walking affords a quality of perception, of interconnected senses, moving through the environment picking up signals, like a conversation. Something becomes available. The world presents itself to us, comes to our attention. What presents itself is not just what is predicted, anticipated, expected, remembered—instead, it is this moment, as in meditation. Walking is a way to experience being in touch with our surroundings.

In familiar or unfamiliar territory, we could set our senses for pick-up, exploration. Thanks to a million years of evolution, we don't have to use a lot of brain cells to pay attention to the act of walking itself. Instead, our attention can be with the space we are moving through/within. Resting in this comfortable, familiar movement, the familiar rhythms, the scenery passing, something is freed, made available. Walking through the world is so essentially, so deeply in us that we can let go into it, which means letting go to being here.

Time today is measured in milliseconds. The automatic response to sound is less than 10 milliseconds. Ears process sounds in 40 milliseconds, faster than the eyes/visual cortex can process an image. Visual processing is significantly slower: it takes 200 milliseconds, one-fifth of a second, for a visual impression to organize into an image that registers on our conscious awareness. *Andante*, at a walking pace, the world presents itself, comes to us, calls us. Walking gives the time for us to go from reactivity to registering, allowing an impression to form.

When I mentioned the 200 milliseconds required for an image to form to my client Jeff, a computer programmer working at a video game company in Boston, he exclaimed, "200 milliseconds!" "Is that a lot or a little?" I asked. He said, "We have six milliseconds to make the whole scene appear on the screen." Hearing that, I realized how many people today—children, too—are being bombarded by a level of stimulation that is far beyond our capacity to process. To allow perception to happen at a more human pace, we may need to pause just a little. Now Jeff and I joke, "Got 200 milliseconds?"

These days, walking is measuring every step in an app. Often, we are walking as fast as we can just to increase our score to get to 10,000. This goal came about as a clever marketing ploy from the creators of the first pedometer in the 1960s. The Japanese company Yamasa Tokei Keiki Co., Ltd. named the pedometer "*Manpo-kei*"—*manpo* means 10,000 steps in Japanese. From a health perspective, 10,000 is an arbitrary number, but it makes a great target for a certain kind of walking (YAMAX, n.d.).

But what if we let go of the way of thinking that chooses an arbitrary goal and measures every step, and, instead, move through the environment at a more human pace, a tempo that allows time to take in what surrounds us? We can trust our sense of balance to run the show, leaving us free for the most important task: encountering the world. Potentially, we can rest in walking—but if we don't surrender, we take our standing (our attitude) with us. Nothing new can be experienced. In this day and age, to find this potential may take practice: the practice of unlearning holding ourselves, unlearning effort. Walking itself might be this practice, which allows us to find how to surrender and free the Where brain. Resting in walking makes a different world available.

Our whole system registers what is before us, around us: a field, not a line, the surroundings, not just what is in front. With the sense of ground and sky, the spine becomes an infinite line, an axis. Then there is no need to close down in front, no doing or task to close us up or close us in. The whole front of the body, even inside, the wet visceral space, is free to respond. It is all being touched, knowing through being touched.

With this attitude, the information pick-up system gets tuned, and we may become available for something new to present itself, for beauty. We could move toward what calls us—to see/be with before labeling, before knowing. Then could we pause, get closer, get intimate with form, shape, texture, impression? That's the capacity that could be tuned, exercised, awoken. This is not an objectifying gaze; instead, could we allow a little space before memory and associations enter, letting ourselves be touched through see/feel eyes, to experience instead of representing?

Feeling the walking that just happens and that includes the surroundings—the balance of perceiving our body and perceiving the world—both supports and frees perception. This balance allows a change in the relationship with environment from me-inside and that-out-there to a tender relationship: ourselves the material on which the impression is made.

Next time you are out walking, try it for yourself.

GETTING OVER YOUR FEET

The physiology that we have been exploring—all that goes into walking—can be expressed in a simple movement such as standing up from our chairs and sitting back down. As we saw with the biped robots, moving from sitting to standing is a complex balancing act. It is a key activity in daily life and a well-known movement practice in somatic traditions such as the Alexander Technique. My understanding of this fundamental movement deepened as Hubert led us in a workshop in Chandolin, Switzerland, in 2008. Balancing, the signals we tune to when orienting, how we use gaze, all enter in. He showed us a way to explore the movement that took it far beyond just a leg strengthening exercise. We can use sitting and standing as a tuning practice, teaching us what to pay attention to, inviting us to notice tension in the toes or the fronts of the shins, for example—subtle signs of being off balance. Then we can carry these new perceptions into walking.

TRY THIS

Here's a way to experience getting over your feet in sitting and standing. It is best to use a bench or chair with a flat, firm seat. Stand up and sit down a few times. What comes to your attention? What do you notice?

Coming into standing is a big change in our base of support, from the chair to the floor. There are many elements, so let's start with our feet. Where does the center of gravity fall on our feet as we come into standing? You can try this with feet parallel or staggered.

And what happens as we sit back down? Do the toes pop off the ground? Do we fall into the chair?

This time, as you sit and stand, adopt the intention to allow your feet and shins to stay soft. Standing and sitting a couple of times, can your feet stay rooted, quiet, free to feel the ground?

Take the time to feel the weight on the feet. At the moment when you want to pull the toes up or grab, that's the moment to stay with the connection into the ground through the feet.

Then starting again, from sitting to standing to sitting.

Where would we want the center of gravity to fall on the feet?

People are given so much misinformation about our feet. Flat feet, hammer toes, pronation—all these issues are considered problems of the feet themselves. Consequently, the solutions proposed are to fix the feet: through stiff orthotics for flat feet, or surgery for hammer toes, or by using constant muscular effort to maintain the foot in supination with the weight on the outside edge to counter pronation.[4] Do these solutions necessarily make sense?

One important element is where and how the weight from above falls into the foot—where the center of gravity falls, so the foot can be a good palpator of the ground and a good spring. Stiff orthotics may not allow natural movement of the joints—the subtalar and the tibiotalar—and thus the flat foot correction can lead to a new problem in the knee, for instance. Hammer toes are often a consequence of habitually landing with weight behind Chopart's joint line—also known as the transverse tarsal joint where the talus and navicular and the calcaneus and cuboid meet. [Figure 5] Why not try a postural intervention before opting for surgery?

Dr. Rolf famously said that flat feet aren't flat feet, but rather flat shins. Once we look at the joint relationships in movement, it's clear that the tibia's small amount of rotation is crucial to the dynamics of the foot. And as for holding our feet in supination to correct a flat foot, how can the foot respond to the ground to push off if it is being held in a position with muscular effort?

These are not foot problems! They are problems of relationship of forces: how the weight from above falls into the foot, and how the foot meets the ground (which is sometimes a floor). Sometimes the foot is sacrificed to fashion footwear like high heels or flipflops, which require a person to grip the toes to hold the shoe on the foot. Some types of footwear can get in the way of the force traveling through the foot and in the way of the foot feeling the ground.

Figure 5: Chopart's joint

On a practical level, there are enormous unintended consequences when we don't pay attention to the moment the weight meets the floor through the feet. We pay in neck and shoulder tension when we recruit these structures to get us out of our chairs. When there is no sense of connection with the floor, the muscles are inadequately nourished, so we pay in increasing weakness and falls. What's missing is not merely muscle strength. What's missing is the perceptual body.

In this chapter, we explored the inheritance of a human biped: from the shape of our bones to the intricate capacities of the vestibular system, we are ready to encounter the world. Our emotional system, responding to what is around us, is part of our movement capacity, not a separate channel. But it's not enough to have the inheritance; we have to learn to wield it, to use it. We need to find practices that hone our abilities and help us experience the relationship between how we feel emotionally and what our movement system is up to. That is the role of embodiment practices, from simply standing and sitting, to exercising our range of visual perception as we will explore in the next embodiment practice.

EMBODIMENT: WHAT AND WHERE IN PRACTICE

Though often neglected in traditional exercise, the quality of our gaze has an impact on movement and stability. We will use the understanding of What and Where gazes that we explored earlier in this chapter in the following sitting and standing exploration. Remember that, ideally, the two gazes work together smoothly like a camera's zoom and wide-angle lens. But sometimes our gaze is stuck.

Sitting on your chair as before, let's start with a local gaze—using the What system first. Let your eyes focus on a point close by, perhaps the floor just in front of you, or focus on a specific part of something you see—the title of a book on the shelf, a detail of the painting on the wall. Keep focusing specifically on that point as you rise from sitting to standing and then return to sitting.

For many of us, engaging foveal vision, the narrow view, could be associated with tension in the front of the shins; the ankles (in particular, the tibiotalar joints) will lose their freedom of movement. Releasing that focus, allowing our gaze to widen, letting our gaze become a receiving gaze, expanding into peripheral vision, to find more freedom in the ankles — can the tibia slide on the talus?

Sitting again: This time allow your gaze to widen to take in the periphery of your room—you are not focusing on a specific object, but rather opening your visual field to take in the whole of your space. With this peripheral gaze, stand and sit again. Notice what you are feeling in your lower legs and ankles now as you stand and sit with peripheral gaze.

Do you experience how a change in gaze, a change in the tuning of perception in relation to our surroundings, can directly influence our biomechanics?

Just a little difference in our center of gravity, how our center of gravity relates to the base of support, can change the freedom of the foot to respond to the floor—for better or worse. Keeping the center of gravity behind Chopart's line, the muscles that travel from shin to foot would have to retain their tension, interfering with the foot's response to the floor. This is much easier to feel in the constrained movement of standing and sitting, and then can be carried over into finding this dynamic relationship in walking.

Of all the things we could pay attention to, how we meet the ground from above and from below may be one of the simplest and most important. Every time we sit down or stand up, every step we take, we could be attending to what Dr. Rolf called "appropriate relationship": how to let gravity work for us. The precise anatomical imagery and biomechanics in Hubert's embodiment experiences that I have shared with you, combined with the perspective of non-doing, can help us connect with the forces in the environment to help life flow more easily. Letting go, instead of holding on.

CHAPTER FOUR

Body in Motion

To open up the question of how we think about movement, this chapter explores Soviet neurophysiologist Nikolai Bernstein's idea of coordinative structure. As Thelen and Gibson argue (Chapter One), our conceptual framework shapes what we do. This chapter travels from Bernstein in Russia to movement scientist Michael Graziano at Princeton University, by way of neurosurgeon Wilder Penfield in Canada. We will include views of the body in ancient Greece and China, all to uncover the origins and limitations of the conventional view of the brain's control of movement. Bernstein's understanding of coordinative structure and Gibson's ecological psychology offer another perspective in which action systems become the functional units and include orientation (how not to fall down) in every action. Along with the language of dynamic systems explored in Chapter One, these perspectives provide language to describe Hubert's approach to embodiment practice.

DEGREES OF FREEDOM

I remember when Hubert began to talk about coordination in 1995. We were having class at a movement studio in Holderness, New Hampshire, for the first time. We were sitting on long, narrow benches in a narrow room. Hubert began to tell us more about his work with breast cancer patients and what he called the structure of coordination.

In his work at the cancer research hospital in Milan, he had seen many people post-surgery, with one missing muscle. For the breast reconstruction, the pectoralis minor, latissimus dorsi, sternocleidomastoid, or rectus abdominis might have been removed by the surgeon. The impact of the surgery on the women's movement capacity depended on how each woman organized her movement in gravity. "If people have good health in the lumbar area, you can cut the rectus," he told us, "but if there is a lack of organization in the back, cutting the rectus turns out to be very problematic." There was an order to the way the women coordinated their movement that could be disrupted by the surgery. In this sense, the pattern of coordination was a kind of structure.

The Russian neurophysiologist Nikolai Bernstein was the first person to describe coordination as a structure. Working in the time of the Iron Curtain, Bernstein (1896–1966) did not become known in the West until shortly after his death when his book *The Coordination and Regulation of Movements* was translated into English (Bernstein, 1967). Coordinated movement is much more complex than the typical image in which we simply give orders to the body from the top down. Each joint has several directions in which it can move. For the brain to control the arm alone would require seven commands for the joints. If there had to be a signal to each arm muscle individually, that would require 26 commands. If the commands were directed at individual motor units, it would require a conservative estimate of 2600 separate commands. That's a lot of variables for the arm alone! It would simply take too long for movement to be coordinated if each element had to be addressed individually. So how does the nervous system manage? In movement science circles, this problem is known as the "degrees of freedom" problem.

Bernstein measured the time it took for a subject to push a button: the time between the signal and the action, also known as *latency*. Pushing a button is a simple movement of one finger using only a few muscles. Bernstein compared that to the amount of time between the starting gun going off and a runner coming out of the starting block into the run—a movement that clearly used many more muscles. Yet the latency, the time from the sound to the beginning of the movement, was the same. It was mysterious.

Bernstein's experiment showed that the nervous system had organized all the parts of the movement into a functional unit, so that only one command was needed both for the simple action of pressing the button and for the complex action of the runner launching out of the starting block. Bernstein named this organized unit "coordinative structure."

The idea of coordinative structure is one answer to how the nervous system resolves the degrees of freedom problem. In movement science terms, creating a functional unit of many parts is called creating a "constraint." Coordinated movement is organized along the same lines as a car's axle. Imagine if each wheel, which can move in three directions in space, were controlled independently. Independent movement would require 12 separate orders to steer the car—quite a challenge. Constraining the movement of the back wheels and putting the axle between the two front wheels is a solution. It limits the number of variables so that the car can be driven with a single command from the steering wheel.

I remember listening to Hubert talk about car wheels and wondering what that had to do with the goals of Rolfing, with improving someone's alignment. What was the significance? I didn't like to think about the body as mechanical, and I didn't like math. To think in terms of mechanics seemed objectifying or dehumanizing. Was I mired in a structural view? Or was I resistant to the mechanical viewpoint because I experienced things emotionally? What did degrees of freedom and coordination have to do with me?

As I sat in the movement studio on the narrow bench, I realized that I had never deeply considered how movement was organized, or that movement had to be organized. My unexamined, unconscious theory seemed good enough: "The brain tells the muscles what to do." Moving just happens. Why would I wonder about it?

MOVEMENT MODELS

For practical purposes, some aspects of physical reality can seem abstract or irrelevant. If we believe the earth is flat, how does that impact us getting to the subway? We can find our way to the subway without an understanding of spacetime curvature, whether the earth is flat or whether it is a round orb in a gravitational field. Similarly, walking happens whether we understand it or not. When people believed that the sun rotated around the earth, before Copernicus, they still went about their daily lives, farmed, lived, and died. Their belief may not have impacted daily life in an obvious way, yet it profoundly affected their imagination: how they saw themselves and how they experienced the world. Our conceptual frameworks, conscious or not, affect how we imagine ourselves, how we approach research questions in science, and they impact perception itself.

On a more mundane level, the conceptual framework we adopt as practitioners affects what we do in practice. Even before Hubert's talk, I already had clues that the "brain tells the muscles what to do" theory wasn't the whole story. If that theory was accurate, then it would be very easy to fix problems of movement: we would just tell the person what to do differently and that would be all there was to it. In my experience, this strategy did not work for my clients or myself. I had also read about the career-ending problems coaches had created trying to improve an athlete's performance by asking for deliberate intervention with just one element of form: asking a runner to hold her arms differently or to change the pattern of the foot strike often led to terrible injuries (Kahn, 2010). Instead of improving things, asking athletes to do any intentional act to control their muscles got in the way of performance and efficiency.

The Roboroach from Chapter One illustrates the limitation of the "brain tells each muscle what to do" theory, too. At first, the engineers assumed they could build a replicated structure and attach wires to simulate the nerves, and it would just go. It's easy to unconsciously assume that the brain plays the muscular system like a pianist plays the piano—one key at a time—but when we stop to think about it, it becomes clear that it can't work this way. Bernstein's recognition of the degrees of freedom problem upended years of thinking about the brain's control of movement.

Ironically, imagining the difficulty of controlling all four wheels of a car independently without an axle can help us begin to imagine a more complex view of human movement. With all the degrees of freedom our segmented bodies provide us with, movement would not be possible if the brain had to control each muscle individually. Understanding by building works: in trying to build mobile robots, biped machines, it becomes obvious that instability, managing the effect of gravity in our terrestrial environment, and perceptual processes are key. In reality for us, our instability is a source of information, not a glitch. We feel where we are because of our disequilibrium, our ongoing conversation with our environment. Yet we think of ourselves with a false image of control, willpower, and effort that is all too easily punctured, yet persists. It's a body image, an idea.

Cortical localization

Where did the perspective of the brain controlling individual muscles come from? We have inherited an oversimplified point of view of the brain's control of movement based on the work of German scientists Fritsch and Hitzig in the 1870s and advanced by Canadian neurosurgeon Wilder Penfield in the 1930s. Popularizations of these researchers' findings gave us the image of movement controlled by specific areas in the brain managing specific muscles.

Fritsch and Hitzig's experiments on dogs, which would not be permitted in current times, are often considered the beginning of modern neuroscience (Graziano, 2018). Their experiments confirmed that electrical stimulation of areas of the dog's cortex elicited twitches in various body areas, illustrating the relationship between the motor cortex and the control of movement. This was the start to the notion of cortical localization—that different brain areas serve specifically different functions. It was a stunning revelation that brain matter mattered to movement in a direct way.

During the 1930s, Wilder Penfield (1891–1976) pioneered groundbreaking surgical techniques to treat severe epilepsy. Prior to surgery, while patients were awake under local anesthesia, Penfield used electrical probes to stimulate various areas of the brain with a short electric pulse of 10 or 20 milliseconds. Unlike the dogs, these patients could talk and were able to describe the sensations and movements they experienced, allowing Penfield to be more precise during the surgery and to develop a detailed map of the sensory and motor regions of the cerebral cortex.

Drawing from Penfield's careful notes, photographs, and sketches from 126 patients operated on between 1928 and 1936, Erwin Boldrey, M.D., created an image of a funny-looking human-like creature, the iconic sensory-motor homunculus that appeared for the first time in publication in 1937 (Penfield & Boldrey, 1937). [Figure 6] The image still shows up in textbooks in modern times: a point-to-point map showing the connection between an area of the body that we feel or move and the corresponding neurons in the primary motor cortex or the primary somatosensory cortex (Catani, 2017). The proportion of each body part in the homunculus corresponds to the amount of cortex dedicated to encoding and processing signals from that part. When neuroscientists use terms like map or representation, they are describing a pattern of neural activity that "stands in" for that part. Each part in the homunculus image was drawn in proportion to the amount of cortical area devoted to controlling or sensing that body area based on Penfield's data, resulting in a distorted human figure with big lips and hands. The larger representations reflect body areas that require more fine motor control and sensory input.

The paper made a big impact on both brain surgery and scientific research. In medicine, it helped show that stimulating specific areas of the brain is a useful way to map brain functions during surgery. In science, it supported the idea that different parts of the brain control specific actions, such as movement, touch, and thinking.

Figure 6: Sensory-Motor Homunculus

This map was considered to be more or less fixed throughout life. Today, the image arising from Penfield's findings is being reevaluated in light of new research. Contemporary researchers are finding that the brain is not organized in a simple mechanistic, top-down way at all, but much more by how we do things in the world. Twenty-first-century neuroscience is helping to create a new image of the moving body, one in which brain and body are integrated with their surroundings as a complex system.

The brain is organized by the world

Research undertaken by Michael Graziano's team took a slightly different tack from Penfield, with dramatic results. All they did was increase the duration of the signal to the same area in the motor cortex as in Penfield's experiment, to half a second. Under this influence, the researchers saw something that astonished them. Instead of muscle twitches, the monkeys made much more complex movements, such as reaching with the hand shaped as if about to grasp, bringing hand to mouth, or bringing the arm up in a ward-off gesture, as if defending from a potential impact. These were functional movements, meaningful actions. The longer signal gave enough time for a natural movement to complete itself in what Graziano called a "behavioral timescale" (Graziano *et al.*, 2002).

In a more recent popular recounting of his research, Graziano described the researchers' surprise during the experiment—and the monkey's, too—as its hand reached out and made motions out of its control. Disconcerted at first, the monkey grabbed its own hand and sat on it. Over time in future experiments, the monkey grew accustomed to the experience and was effectively distracted by a steady supply of grapes. But for the researchers who had discovered this extraordinary phenomenon by mistake, it was cataclysmic (Graziano, 2018). Based on nearly 120 years of research, Graziano did not expect to be able to evoke a complex action linking muscles of arm, hand, and mouth from a single location in the motor area of the brain where the electrodes had been placed. His data challenged many of the century-old assumptions about how the brain organizes movement: that it is built up of simple components and organized in a hierarchy. Although it might be tidy to imagine each neuron or group of neurons controlling a particular muscle or joint, or clear demarcations between sensory areas and motor areas, it's not an accurate representation of what goes on in the brain. Instead, Graziano's findings suggest an image of a brain that is a complex network organized by living in the world.

Researchers such as Graziano suggest that the brain may not relate to the body as parts, but to the world through action. That means that movement patterns, not muscles, are the functional "unit." For the monkey, reaching for food and gestures of self-protection are basic functional movement patterns, the actions necessary for a monkey to live in the world. The motor cortex seems to be organized in terms of movement categories, meaningful actions that are part of the animal's—our—everyday movement repertory.

APPLYING SCIENCE TO PRACTICE: WEIGHT TRAINING

How does a change in our understanding of how the brain organizes movement, from a point-to-point correspondence between the motor cortex and the muscle to the perspective of functional movements organized by our activities in the world, impact our everyday life? How would it apply to our approach to exercise, for example? The older model of the motor cortex "talking" to each individual muscle fits with an idea of strengthening individual muscles. But with the suggestion that the motor cortex is actually organized for functional movements, how would our idea of how to improve movement change? Will strengthening individual muscles automatically lead to better movement?

One of my clients owned a roofing company. He had been hauling heavy materials up onto roofs since he was a youngster. He would laugh at his younger helpers who were able to bench-press hundreds of pounds but could not haul a bag of tar up onto a roof or would tire after a couple of hours' work. For those young people, the strength manifesting in the gym was nowhere to be found during the workday.

Is it even possible to strengthen one muscle at a time? When people come in to see me, they often say there is something wrong with their hamstrings, their trapezius, or some other particular muscle. Do muscles go rogue on their own and become individually dysfunctional? Or are they part of a moving system, in which the problem is in the pattern of movement and not in the individual muscles themselves? Could we even get into trouble stretching or strengthening any one area out of context? This was suggested in 2009 as Major League Baseball stars over-strengthened their knees after injuries and ended up with hip problems (Schmidt, 2009). To promote a healthy movement system, it may not make sense to focus on one joint at a time.

Along with Bernstein's work on the structure of coordination, Graziano's research suggests that strengthening muscles independently of meaningful actions may not lead to usable movement skill. While we were working on the Physical Intelligence project at MIT, Noah Riskin, the gymnastics coach, pointed out pulley devices embedded in the floor of the Cambridge campus's original gym—exercise machines from the late 1800s. In contrast to the now-popular Nautilus machines that strengthen muscles group by group, Noah noted that the machines were designed to imitate the movements that the inventor used while working on the farm where he grew up, such as threshing and hoeing.

A useful analogy is to think of muscles as an alphabet. Out of context, there is very little meaning in a letter. A simple action, such as flexing the forearm, is like a word. Advanced readers no longer read letters at all: we grasp a word or even a sentence in one glance. In movement, a functional relationship is like a sentence: that's where the meaning of the movement is conveyed. The meaning is a life-supporting action, a function in the world, like eating, defending, et cetera. Our movements are organized in terms of their goal. We don't have to micromanage our muscles in order to accomplish functional actions.

The need to manage instability and the use of coordinated movement sequences to meet functional goals—reaching for an apple, pushing a shopping cart—applies to us just as it does to the monkeys in the experiment described above and the robots described earlier. Structures of coordination have to include the pre-movements that allow us to orient ourselves in space, to know which way is up, which way is down, and to keep our balance. No matter what our particular vocation, the movements we repeat the most organize orientation so that we can perceive and make sense of the world. Orientation also supports our other most repeated movements: the movements of breath and the movements of walking.

No matter what action we perform with a weight, or in the course of daily life, the rest of our system is busy with the task of making sure we don't fall over, while keeping our head oriented and our gaze able to explore the world (Reed, 1982).

Nested into any functional movement is the importance of maintaining our balance. Strengthening each unit independently (strong biceps, strong triceps, et cetera) may not be as valuable as strengthening the capacity to keep our balance while doing a variety of actions. At the very least, this is an argument for using free weights instead of machines to increase strength. In weight-training circles, the importance of including balance has caught on. Instead of circuit training muscles in an assembly line—one muscle group at a time—functional movements are coming back into fashion. Movements are practiced in multiple dimensions: lifting a sandbag like luggage from the floor, putting it over head, as we do on trains and planes, bringing it back down; picking up the sandbag on one side and moving it across the body to the other side. During all these movements, the dynamic activity of stabilizing to prevent the momentum from knocking us over happens without our thinking about it.

Beyond deliberate exercise, our bodies are shaped by the movements we do most frequently. When I see a person's body, the shape reveals something: does this person spend most of her time working out or lying on the couch? Playing piano, or guitar, or video games? Figure skating or speed skating? All lead to different body shapes. And there is another possible reading: our bodies also can show what we avoid—the movements we do not allow ourselves.

THE INTERPLAY BETWEEN SCIENCE AND CULTURE: THE HISTORY OF MUSCLE

Research such as Graziano's is fairly new and has mostly been performed on rats, cats, and monkeys. It will take many years before we can state with certainty how it applies to human beings. What is clear is that we are going to have to let go of some of our fixed ideas about brain organization and willpower as the way to manage our body's movements.

Oddly, in the case of Graziano's discoveries, it was not only technological innovation (surface stimulation vs micro electrodes) that made new information available. Graziano speculates that the desire to find simplicity in the map of the motor cortex influenced the way research was conducted from 1870 to 2000 (Graziano, 2018, p.69). It was so appealing to envision each individual neuron cleanly corresponding to a single pathway triggering a single set of muscles, the way each key of a piano lifts the damper off a single string and allows a single note to be struck. When anything more complex happened, such as more neurons getting involved, the researchers shortened the timing of the electrical signal to avoid them. Graziano writes, "In effect, scientists treated the widespread connections of the motor cortex as a kind of annoying experimental artifact because it didn't suit the prevailing concept of how the motor system worked" (Graziano, 2018, p.72). Scientists themselves are always embedded in a cultural context that influences the experiments they choose and the phenomena they observe. Researchers in the 19th and early 20th centuries considered the interconnections in the nervous system "noise." Over a hundred years later, exhausted by a perspective that has cut us up and cut us off from the world and each other, we are hungry for interconnectedness. But you have to know where to look for a new perspective to find it in research fields. James Gibson, Edward Reed, Esther Thelen, and Michael Graziano, among others, are reaching past the mechanistic tradition to open Western thinking up to a more complex view.

Popular conception has not yet caught up. Our common ideas about how we move—muscle engines driven by a top-down brain—are a product of a mechanistic paradigm. We are preoccupied by muscle strength and muscle mass. And the value that goes with it, as we have explored in previous chapters, is "mind over matter": the mind as dictator over the body. Bulging biceps and washboard abs acquired through sheer willpower are images of the body from popular culture. These images affect our sense of self: we imagine we should be dominating our bodies to achieve the right look. Effort is valued over responsiveness.

It is easy to forget that our ideas of "good body" are images based in culture, not simple facts. Despite their predominance today, the importance of muscles in the imagination of the body is a fairly recent historical development. In Shigeshisa Kuriyama's beautiful book *The Expressiveness of the Body* (2002), the author makes this point in the chapter entitled "Muscularity and Identity." Comparing ancient Greek and Chinese medicine, Kuriyama describes a time in both cultures when "muscles" were almost completely ignored. The Greeks saw rippling sinews and flesh. Their heroes were moved by the gods, not by their own power. For the

Chinese, what moved was the subtle "mo"—not exactly pulses, perhaps conduits of flowing qi—which could be described in terms such as floating or sunken, hollow or hidden e.g., (Kuriyama, 2002, pp.98–99). These cultures had other ideas about how a body came into motion. The body was moved; it was part of a mysterious larger picture, not an engine for an individual identity. Muscles did not come to Western attention until the first and second centuries CE, not only because of anatomical dissection, but in conjunction with a developing notion of personal will. This worldview adopted muscle as "the organ of voluntary motion" (Kuriyama, 2002, p.144).

As it was for the Chinese and the Greeks, so it is for us: science exists at any given time within a cultural frame that holds certain values, looks for them in the world, and finds them. History tells us that there are fashions in science. Cultural influences establish values which carry over into our approach to research, and most of these remain unconscious. According to George Lakoff, cognitive linguist, it is unlikely that we can think without a frame of reference, so the best we can manage is to try to be somewhat aware of the frames we are holding (Lakoff, 2012).

EMBODIMENT AS AN IMAGINATIVE ACTION

Where in today's culture is there room for the perceptual body, the body experienced as an ongoing relationship with place? I find myself asking this question often. The neuroscience explored in this chapter may allow us to imagine ourselves differently—what Gaston Bachelard called "an imaginative act" (see Orientation: How to Read This Book). We can see a different image, one in which we are organisms inextricably interrelated with our environment. The difference in imagining (taking a different point of view, model, or framework) leads to a different kind of embodiment practice. We need to pay attention to more than the shape of our bodies and how we look in the mirror. We have explored how every movement includes staying upright, oriented in our environment, and how good coordination involves more than just muscular strength. The neuroscience we have considered in these sections suggests that tuning into the pre-movements that support stability will be especially effective because they precede, and shape, support, or limit, every other movement we do.

This understanding was reflected in how we explored embodiment in workshops with Hubert. For example, in the *Stick work* practice discussed in the Introduction, we were not lifting a heavy weight to build strength and challenge our arms or legs, but rather using imagination—imagining a stick that could float—to trigger core support, which would make the movement easier. This approach produced a more coordinated movement than following a direction to just lift our arms up. The movement referenced the world of actions such as reaching or lifting, while at the same time we became followers and listeners to the movement instead of commanders.

Our quality of attention is part of the pre-movement, the preparation for action. Instead of concentrating on lifting or pushing, we can put our attention on the meeting—the contact, the connection—between our hands and the stick, between our feet and the floor. And surprisingly, the actions of reaching or pushing improve as a result of our change in focus. We can hone the skill of tuning in to the most useful information for our action, rather than the end in itself.[1]

Throughout the chapters in Part I, you have been introduced to much of the theory that supports an approach to movement practice based in dynamic systems and ecological psychology. Like the tuna, we can use the forces available in our terrestrial environment to power our movement. The affordances of earth and gravity and horizon give our eyes and our vestibular system useful information. We can learn to use the information supplied by gravity and our inherited structures, such as the springs, levers, and receptors of our feet and limbs, and also to include the contribution of the fluid system, fascia, and connective tissue, as well as muscle power (Bordoni *et al.*, 2019).

We also include our perceptual systems. To help change the patterns of coordination, the sequences of our movements and muscle synergies, we need to reach the pre-movement level—pre-movements that help us orient and stabilize, prepare and initiate action in a given context. Images are one tool we can use to change our movements. In the sitting and standing embodiment, we reach a level at which our physical experience and our emotional experience can be intertwined in unexpected ways. In Chapter Three, we saw how the particular gaze we use can be related to our emotional state—whether gaze is free to move comfortably between focal and peripheral or stuck in one way of looking, for instance. The narrowed gaze from overuse of focal vision may have a direct impact on our ankle joint, as you may have experienced in the sitting and standing segment of the embodiment practice in the previous chapter. Through this chain of events—quality of gaze leading to unintended muscular tensions—the efficiency of many movements such as walking or running can be impacted. For each one of us, our personal way of organizing physical and emotional dimensions enters our way of managing in a gravitational field (Mulla & Keir, 2023).

TRY THIS

Bringing all this new information with us, let's go back to the movements of *Stick work* once again. You can use a thick branch or a closet dowel or even a broom handle—ideally a natural material or something that feels good.

Holding the stick in both hands with your arms hanging in front of you at ease, let yourself notice where you and the stick are touching. Notice the place of contact—the two-way process: you are touching the stick and being touched by the stick at the same time. Notice the feeling of the floor under your feet, and the sense of your surroundings.

Now, let the stick begin to...as if...float up...and let your hands follow it.

Imagine it is floating up and you are hanging from it. Spend some time with this imagining—feeling a little pulled up by the stick and a little hanging—a gentle tug of war.

Now the stick is becoming a heavy weight, pulling you over into a partial forward bend. Spend a little time feeling the pull of the floor and the pull of the stick.

With a sense of the stick as heavy, begin to come back to your starting point, allowing each pair of vertebrae to link into a system as you stand up.

You can go through this process several times.

How has your experience changed since the movement was introduced at the start of the book?

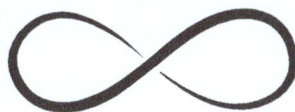

As we will explore in the chapters ahead, the deepest habits, common to us all, are habits of perception, how we take in the world, and habits of keeping our balance, how we organize ourselves in gravity. Perception is the start button that allows a movement sequence to unfold. Changes in perception allow changes in our coordination. Perceptual and imaginative processes allow us to tune orientation and coordinative structures.

PART II

EXPRESSING

CHAPTER FIVE

Cultural Body

As we have seen in the previous chapters, current science supports a more sophisticated point of view than that of a body of muscle bossed around by a brain, disconnected from the environment. Yet that image persists in popular culture. How does the image of being a machine or a collection of parts impact us? Is it just a simple choice between two equally valuable ways of modeling our complexity? What kind of trouble can arise from the images we hold of ourselves as bodies?

BODY WORLDS

Shortly after the MIT project in 2006, a daring exhibit called *Body Worlds* arrived at the Museum of Science in Boston (Body Worlds, 2024). "Groundbreaking Anatomical Exhibit! Real Human Bodies on Display!" read the advertising. Controversy surrounded the exhibition. *Body Worlds* makes exhibits out of dead people, the critics wrote, desecrating their bodies and disrespecting death itself (Collier, 2010). Nonetheless, curious and interested people flocked to the show. Somewhat reluctantly, I was among them.

When I first studied anatomy in the 1980s as an alternative medical practitioner, it wasn't easy to get a chance to do an actual dissection. Through a friend in medical school, I gained access to an anatomy laboratory—a rare privilege at that time. There, cadavers that had been preserved with formaldehyde were kept carefully wrapped on large metal gurneys. We exposed only a small part of the body at a time, for the most part keeping their faces covered. There was a sense of reverence in approaching them.

Body Worlds was different. These corpses were on display, posing and peering. Frozen in time, eyeballs glaring, an upright archer held a bow

with an outstretched arm. Careful dissection unveiled the muscular structure beneath the skin. A horse reared, defying gravity. Its rider, muscles
exposed, clung to the horse's mane. Two dancers embraced, captured in
a leap. The spine of one was pulled apart from the rest of its body.

Body Worlds' producers proudly proclaimed that over 9000 volunteers
had agreed to be preserved in this way. The website explained that the
unusual poses "allow the visitor to relate the plastinate [the preserved
cadaver] to his or her own body" (Körperwelten, 2024). But I felt a deep
sense of dismay. Here, through miraculous modern technology, we were
invited to look under the skin—but these bodies were literally dead and
completely inert despite their "realistic attitudes." No feelings, no breathing, no moving.

The exhibit conveyed the idea that bodies are an assemblage of parts
and positioning, a skeleton scaffolding with muscles put on like clay. One
model literally held its own flayed bag of skin, like a removable wrapper.
Circulation was rendered as static and able to be artfully separated from
the whole, an inert red cloud of capillaries. What did these bodies have
to do with my actual experience of being embodied? Here the dead body
was posed as a living one, and what had been flesh was literally turned
into an object.

Along with the ghoulish thrill, the exhibit was a technological marvel.
Its creator, Gunther von Hagens, had developed a technique he called
"plastination": by replacing the body's fluids with resins and elastomers, he
was able to preserve the dead flesh and prevent decomposition. Working
as an anatomy assistant, von Hagens had seen a kidney sample encased
in a plastic square and conceived the idea of putting the plastic in the
flesh itself to expose the sample. The technique not only gave the corpse
"rigidity and permanence," but also allowed it to be sculpted, turned into
an action figure. Plastination replaced the body's intricate interactions
with place, its responsiveness and relationship with the environment.

Although the fibers and organs were exposed for all to see, for me they
did not reveal what really matters. The sense of embodiment that Hubert
had helped me cultivate over 15 years was decidedly *not* represented at
Body Worlds. Body, to me, is warm and full of feeling. Body, to me, is a
way of being in touch—with sounds, smells, and sensations, with breath,
with change.

The plastinates I was encouraged to relate to were not responsive to
their surroundings at all. Contrary to the marketing materials, I do not
want to see myself that way! There was no exchange going on. Even a dead

body is still interacting under normal circumstances: it is in a process of decay. Plastination took the body out of the realm of organic material. The figures stayed upright and held poses while completely insensate, as if perceiving and sensing could be separated from the body in action.

This attitude of separation goes far beyond anatomy, all the way to our sense of self and the complex problem of body image. Like the robot bodies in *The Six*, the *Body Worlds* exhibit reflected our vulnerable, impermanent selves in a mirror of permanence and invulnerability.

The action poses and the muscular layers on display imply that feelings, sensations, and perceptions are irrelevant or at least a separate dimension from the body in action. The displays in the *Body Worlds* exhibit seemed to me to be perpetuating an important, unexamined assumption: the actual body is *animate*, while the bodies in *Body Worlds* are objects. An actual living being has no on/off switch. We are essentially feeling, perceiving, essentially in motion and responding to the immediate context.

No one around me seemed to have this reaction. People were understandably fascinated by seeing under the skin, but they did not seem to be relating the plastinates to their own bodies. For some, the plastinates were like sculptures, remarkable works of art. For others, to see under the skin was like looking under the hood of a car to see the engine or taking the cover off a computer to reveal the boards and circuits inside. But what did this have to do with our own embodiment?

Like the cerebral mystique, *Body Worlds* presents an example of a powerful image or idea of body that exists in our culture. Many people—including the ones that I encounter in my practice as a Rolfer—have learned to see themselves as machines or objects. Exhibits like *Body Worlds*, along with fashion magazines, workout attitudes, and many medical practices, reinforce an image of the body with component parts which malfunction. The living, perceptual body—feeling, moving, and relating to gravity—is entirely eclipsed. How is this attitude affecting us?

PRACTICAL IMPLICATIONS OF THE BODY-MACHINE IMAGE

CLIENT STORY: MARTA

A new client, Marta, came in, referred by her colleague who was happy with the results from coming to see me. A small, dark-haired woman, an engineer who spent hours at her computer, she hoped to find relief for her back pain. As I observed her standing in my office, I could see the habitual hunch: though upright, it was as if she were still sitting at the computer as far as her chest and shoulders were concerned.

To see how a person organizes themselves in gravity requires looking past the symptom to see the physics of the situation. Marta said she was a runner, but I could see it would be hard for her back to manage the ground forces that push up in running. The holding in her upper body almost prevented the weight from reaching the ground. Was this guarding against putting weight into the painful part of her back, or was it leading her into back pain in the first place? I wouldn't know until we got to work.

I started by addressing the hunch. With Marta lying on her back, I helped her tune in to the support from the table through words and through touch so that her muscles could let go of their holding pattern. But when I began to work with her feet, she said, "As long as we focus on the back—that's what is important to me." I often notice this attitude: many clients come in with an image of the body as a collection of malfunctioning parts. In this view, the symptom is the only problem, the part that needs fixing. To help her see beyond this cultural myth of the body, I explained that our back is adapting to the forces from above (the weight of the chest/arms/head) and to the forces from below (the push-off when our feet meet the ground). We could imagine the back as a traffic rotary, or roundabout: cars are coming from multiple directions, and the rotary has to allow them to flow through. Back pain is often a relationship issue: the forces from above and below aren't working together effectively. To help a particular place in the back, we often need to take a bigger view and see the physics of the whole system.

Beyond materials

Physics, however, is only one of the influences on a human being. Efficiently using the materials of our joints and flesh to best advantage is only one facet of our movement experience. We don't always care about efficiency in movement because conserving our mechanical energy isn't as vital to us as it is to the tuna we encountered in Chapter One. There is more to the body and to movement than mechanics.

Another influence is emotional: the need to feel as secure as possible might mean limiting the degrees of freedom in movement as much as possible. In learning to ski, for example, the response to the unfamiliar sliding, to the risk of being out of control, is usually to stiffen up, to limit motion at the joints. A frightened animal or person may curl in on themself, seeking protection and stability. The easiest movement, mechanical efficiency, may be overridden by the important need to feel secure.

The social context is another factor that shapes what movements are and are not acceptable, efficiency be damned. For example, in some cultures, freedom of movement is a social taboo for a woman. I remember a client who had worked in the Peace Corps in Kurdistan and told me that while living in a small rural village, she had to change her posture completely to avoid unwanted attention. Not looking up, keeping her chest down, avoiding eye contact, and moving quickly to get to a safe place became her way of life, constraining her body. In other cultures, men may be taught to avoid hip movement, leading to a restriction in every step. Neither robot nor tuna change their movement patterns based on social pressures they experience, but these pressures are a key factor to consider for human beings. Over the course of a series of sessions with a client, together we can explore the impact that social constraints may be having on movement patterns as their individual story unfolds.

What are the unintended consequences of the relentless images of body-machine with its replaceable parts, or action without perception as in the *Body Worlds* plastinates? Can holding these images of our own embodiment be harming us?

WHAT IS A RELIABLE BODY?

I was not the only one experiencing dismay at the images of the body at *Body Worlds* and in our culture. I found my concerns echoed by Susie Orbach, a British psychotherapist known for treating Diana, Princess of Wales, in her struggle with bulimia. Referring to the *Body Worlds* exhibit in her 2009 book, *Bodies*, Orbach wrote that such exhibits "alert us to a pervasive cultural dysmorphia. They tell us we've lost the plot where bodies are concerned" (Orbach, 2009, p.176). What did she mean?

Like the plastinates in the *Body Worlds* exhibit, *body* has become a kind of product to be exercised, to look right, to be worked out, to be managed. Orbach relates this attitude to the post-industrial age. She says that we labor at the gym now to create the look of the laborers in the field of years past. But it isn't just how we look; it's that we have lost touch with what bodies are for. The body has become a commodity, an object, instead of an experience. This body image is seen from the outside. Our felt experience is transformed into a visual representation, and we literally lose touch. We become prisoners of the mirror, able only to know ourselves through distorted reflections.

For example, let's see how the problem applies to posture. My clients often tell me that they catch sight of their terrible posture in reflections from shop windows: "My head is so far forward; my chest is so sunken. Can you straighten me out?" Rolfing Structural Integration, my profession, is known as deep fascial manipulation that realigns the body. People come into my office every day thinking a well-aligned body means looking straight. Whether they have been practicing yoga, going to tai chi, visiting the chiropractor or looking in the mirror while lifting weights, good form means things should line up. There is some legitimacy to the idea of alignment. But where is it misleading?

In the mirror of the shop window, my clients see a still body, a moment in time. They see an image, a visual instead of a felt experience. They think of that image and try to create good posture—another image but this time held up through effort. It's the plastinated body but in real life: putting oneself in what seems visually like the right position and holding it. Since as living beings we do not have the "benefits" of plastination, for us to hold a posture takes enormous effort that actually interferes with the body in motion.

Stand up straight!

How many times have you heard that command and pulled yourself out of your slouch with a lot of effort, only to find yourself collapsed again a moment later? Well-intentioned mothers, grandmothers, coaches, and army sergeants all learned this idea somewhere: shoulders back, chest out. This is supposed to be good posture, something you *hold*. That approach may work for a moment, while your mom is watching or while you're waiting for the camera to click, but it's likely that the next minute, you will be back in your familiar, habitual slouch.

Or, worse yet, you could get good at holding. A Pilates instructor who came to me told me she was instructed to hold her shoulder blades pinned together—that was the idea of good posture that was imposed on her at one Pilates studio. She was told that when she raised her arm, her shoulder blades should not move at all. This is a misguided interpretation of biomechanics,[1] but it is a good example of how body image and lack of accurate information lead us to try to control our posture. This is a terrible, unsustainable effort that eventually leads to joint problems—problems that could be avoided if we tried *less*.

A very different result arises when we find alignment as a sense of our weight resting into the ground and the capacity for our senses to take in the environment. There is no mirror reflecting in this approach: instead, it's an actual feeling of solidity and support. Unfortunately, the admonition to stand up straight doesn't capture the physical reality of effective organization in gravity.

As Orbach said, we have "lost the plot where bodies are concerned" (Orbach, 2009, p.176). 2018 was the 40th anniversary of Orbach's book *Fat Is a Feminist Issue*. Orbach reported feeling appalled that her book—originally published in the 1970s—was still in print. Far from getting better, she expressed, the only thing that had changed was that hating our bodies had become a problem more or less equally shared by men and women.

Made not born

In her 2009 book, *Bodies*, Orbach tried to sound the alarm about the damage being done to us all by the misrepresentations of the cultural body. She described how each week we are inundated with 5000 or more images that have been airbrushed and retouched 30 to 40 times. With the social media of 2025, today this number must have multiplied a hundred-fold. We develop warped ideas of what we are supposed to look like, while at the same time being reminded that looks are what matter most. Plastic surgery is a huge business, growing by one billion dollars each year. Beyond Botox injections and the tummy tuck, Orbach gives the example of Chinese women using cosmetic tape to hold their eyelids open to create a wider eye shape, refreshing it several times over the course of a night's date. Taping eyelids may seem innocent enough, but Orbach also recounts horrific surgeries such as those of women in Fiji who have their legs broken and lengthened with metal bars to look more Western. The devastating consequences of racism reflected in idealized beauty standards based on white bodies add to the unrealistic beauty standards imposed on women of all races. Over a decade later, chillingly, cosmetic surgery apps are marketed to little girls as games in which they anticipate surgeries they will have later in life. People are taught that the body is an object, one that needs improvement, like a house that needs renovation.

The clients Orbach describes in *Bodies* have eating disorders or are distraught about their sex lives, their children, relationships, or jobs. They also perceive something not right about their bodies. Culturally, we tend to think of these problems as psychological, but Orbach helps us see that "not quite right" exists in a blended psychophysical domain.

Orbach's perception mirrors my own experience working with clients with chronic pain, joint problems, and bad posture—so-called physical problems. My clients speak to me of their problems in a way that is very much like talking to a mechanic about a car. "I have a bad back," they tell me. "There is something wrong with my knee." Like Marta, who came to me about her back pain, they identify the problem as a part that has gone wrong. Sometimes they say they wish the part could be removed and replaced. By the time they come to me, they have often seen a doctor and been through a series of tests. They are accustomed to talking to doctors about their body parts, and that's the way they see themselves. Orbach calls this attitude "bodily disenfranchisement." The body is a malfunctioning machine. But could there be another way? What would it mean to see the body as a living organism, with its own kind of needs, its own kind of order?

My clients may have had surgeries or accidents, but many times the cause of their pain is a mystery. Often, they have diligently exercised, doing what the physical therapist prescribed, and carefully monitored their diets, and yet their bodies aren't working right. They feel tight, uncomfortable. Their bodies are giving them trouble. They can't do what they want—for example, keep exercising or work for long hours at the computer. So much for effort: the body defies their will. They don't know what to do, and they feel frustrated. They may also feel confused or hopeless or angry. They feel bad about loss of control and of the positive self-image of being someone who knows what they want and can get it.

After all, we are not taught what it means to be a body: a living organism. In the service of body image, the actual needs of the flesh-and-blood body-organism are often ignored or misunderstood. Although we learn about evolution in school, we don't ask ourselves what it means to live with the force of gravity, to live as other animals do, reacting and responding to our environment. We don't think of posture as an orientation to our environment. We only think of it as standing up straight.

Embodying anxiety

Beyond biology and evolution, our posture reflects our personal feelings as well as cultural influences. To get at this complexity, we need a different term than "body." Orbach chooses "embodiment"—in this case, to describe the living experience of body. She calls it "a place to live from." Echoing French philosopher Simone de Beauvoir's famous statement "One is not born, but rather becomes, a woman" (De Beauvoir, 1949/1956, p.273), Orbach says the same of "body": we are made, not born. In other words, our experience of body is not just genetics. It is shaped by our culture and through our family. It is inculcated and passed on in the way we are touched and fed and clothed from birth.

These days, Orbach wrote, we are receiving an embodiment of anxiety: mothers may pass on their body insecurity to their children through their touch, their words, and the example of their own movement and posture. Throughout her book and in interviews, Orbach refers to an unstable body, an unreliable body, a need to recorporealize. She says that her patients often lack a comfortable sense of embodiment. Their exercise regimes, surgeries, and diets are part of a search to get a body that feels stable, secure, and reliable. In my office, I see the same search for a stable body: some of my clients adopt rigid postures as a way to find a measure of emotional stability. Yet the strategies imposed on the body in the name of an unacknowledged need for emotional security don't allow the adaptability required of a moving organism.

Orbach and I both see the impact of body distress on people at an emotional level. Although Orbach is a psychoanalyst by training, she makes an important point: we shouldn't assume the body is in trouble because of the mind, because we shouldn't assume that the mind comes first. Orbach writes:

> Always situating the origins of the distress in the mind is often not an accurate or sufficient form of understanding. It is an easy kind of analysis, but it can miss the severity of the dis-ease that pertains to the body as a body. Taking on the idea of the symptomatic body as a signal of a body that is struggling to express itself and its needs, or even to exist, is more challenging and it is an important place to start. (Orbach, 2009, p.76)

When I read Orbach's words, they resonated with what I had experienced through getting Rolfed as a 17-year-old. The body has something to express. It isn't always what we imagine or what we want. What is the body saying? In the usual meaning of psychosomatic, the symptom reflects an emotional or mental problem. The mind comes first. But what is the larger view of psychosomatic? What is the full voice of the body? What does embodiment mean?

To address some of the concerns she described in *Bodies*, Susie Orbach took action, working with the Dove corporation to create the Real Body advertising campaign, which features women and girls with many different looks openly describing their insecurities about their bodies. The ads push back against the idealized body promoted in our time and open the door to a deeper conversation about body image. We need to challenge these assumptions, but that's not enough. We have to go beyond just changing the commercials to which we are exposed to ask ourselves: What is the root of our insecurity? What are bodies for? Many questions follow: How do we meet the emotional body? And how do we uncover and sustain a reliable body? What is needed to change the images we have of the body itself, our understanding of embodied experience?

CULTIVATING A RELIABLE BODY

Hubert's approach to movement responded to these questions and concerns. From the very first image of Van Gogh's "First Steps," Hubert's point of view was never objectifying. There were no exercises to perform mechanically. How different from the usual repetitive motions that are prescribed in many settings! Instead, each experience was phenomenological: from the first-person perspective. How I made contact with the world around me, the objects, the people, the space, sky and ground, what I noticed, where I put my attention, all mattered to the movement—I, the experiencer, was included. What I felt and how I worked with my own perceptions were what mattered, not how I looked in the mirror or to another person. Grounding ourselves in our own experience is vital in allowing us to find a reliable body.

Hubert's work was unusual in the somatic world. Anatomical specificity and directing our sensory attention were in the service of dynamic actions and relationship: walking, pushing, increasing our stability and sense of security and agency. He avoided leading us into long periods of lying down, and instead kept our attention in the present moment, not "entranced." Each embodiment practice developed our capacity for comfortable relationship with another person or object in the world of action. To find our own standing, we need to include our relationship to gravity, our capacity for action, and also our connection with the Other.

Even with yoga and meditation, which are often thought of as spiritual practices, it is easy to become focused on results at the expense of how we accomplish them, the ends rather than the process. Unfortunately, the very effort involved in trying to *make* something happen may work against good coordination. F. M. Alexander coined the expression "end-gaining" to give a name to this attitude.

Alternatively, what Hubert would call "choosing good information"— useful information the environment provides—usually means starting by seeking better support in relation to gravity. When we find that support ongoingly, we are able to feel stronger for less effort, to adapt and respond to different situations. As we practiced with *Pushing the chair* in Chapter Two, the ability to find our own center in relationship is simultaneously a physical and an expressive act. The physical act is to find support that leads to better mechanics. At the same time, the support allows some independence when we communicate with an Other, rather than merging. This capacity creates the foundation for a more reliable body.

In our embodiment practices, we can practice comfortable personhood, exploring relationship, as described in the *Embodiment* sections— *Stick work*, *Waiting to be called*, *Pushing the chair*—and build security as we do in *Getting over our feet*. When we seek a skillful stability, it serves our whole being, mechanics, emotions, and sense of self. This is a worthy alternative to contrast with the cultural image of the perfect body.

EMBODIMENT: WHAT PREVENTS ME?

Hubert's approach to embodiment practice invites us to look for what is getting in the way instead of trying to make something happen. It is common, in our actions, to focus on the *doing*. We contract muscles, create tension, and try very hard to do a move the right way. In the embodiment practice that follows, we are invited to start differently, by letting go. Hubert sometimes borrowed the phrase *via negativa*, from the Latin—the study of what *not* to do. The approach that starts with letting go has its roots in many ancient philosophical traditions (Fagenblat, 2017). Here we apply it to a movement. Instead of working with effort, we are invited to find an easier way that will still offer strength and responsiveness, not rigid adherence to the familiar way. We are cultivating a new way: starting by letting go.

Let's go back to sitting and standing and continue our exploration with Orbach's questions in mind. Imagine we are doing this movement together, the two of us or with a group. Remember that as we go from sitting to standing, we are allowing our weight to transfer so we can find good support through the meeting of our weight, our feet, and the floor. We used Chopart's line (discussed in Chapter Three) as a reference for this. What prevents the weight from getting over Chopart's line may be more than just a mechanical issue. We may find that some muscular holding in some area of the body is getting in the way of the weight getting over our feet. Something may need to let go.

For instance, what if we start by sliding forward on the chair, letting the fold at our hips deepen, and pour the weight into the ground before standing up, not concerning ourselves with how we look to each other, but instead how the ground feels under our feet? We want to turn away from the mirror into finding authentic support.

As we allow this movement, some holding in the back of the rear end or the pelvic floor may release, or we may become aware of the holding there. Does it feel safe in this moment to let the holding go?

Another element we can experiment with is how our spine/trunk is participating: how does the feeling of pouring the weight through our feet into the ground change if we let our hands rest on our knees, elbows pointing away from the center, and let our spine extend? To find extension, we might ask for letting go of the front surface of the body, the tension that pulls the chest and pelvis together in the front.

Or our emotional response to a situation could be involved:

What if we reach with hands and arms, as if there were a friend across the room waiting for our embrace, and allow that to help with the standing up?

Any of these dimensions—are they getting in the way or can they participate in making this movement easy by letting go of unnecessary tension?

Each of these movements can be evocative. Feelings and even memories or associations may come to the surface as we explore different kinds of expression in our movements. The setting has to feel safe and supportive to allow this kind of expansion. Whether as a client or a practitioner, we need a framework that includes both the mechanics of moving in gravity as well as our human experience.

Many of us who are drawn to approaches like Hubert's find the cultural image of body/object and the disconnection between this body image and our felt experience to be deeply disquieting. Those concerns led us to somatic practices. But unless we also look at the cultural paradigm surrounding body, there is a danger that the somatic practices will fall into the existing categories: bodily experience subsumed by the mind; yoga turned into an Olympic event; tai chi forms practiced as repetitive choreography. We want to see embodiment as psychophysical—not two separate dimensions. How would a new model of integration be described in practice and in theory? As we will explore in the next chapter, Hubert presented us with exactly the right ingredients to allow this integration.

CHAPTER SIX

A New Model of Integration

This chapter begins with a client story illustrating the way a physical symptom like a knee problem may be related to more than the structure of the knee itself. The symptoms that manifest in one joint may be more effectively addressed when we consider the bigger field that includes coordination, perception, and meaning making.

At a workshop in 2000, Hubert presented us with a framework that explored how each of these domains is a form of structure or habit; and how each can be an entry point to opening new possibilities in the whole system. This framework gives language to a new model of integration in which the body's mechanics are fundamentally interwoven with our perceptual habits and our symbolic associations.

CLIENT STORY: MAGIC WORDS

A petite senior citizen who taught elementary school for many years, Carol had been coming for sessions with me for a few months to address her posture and her knee problems.

Carol did Iyengar yoga with a teacher who was very precise: by Carol's report, the teacher called the class members' attention first to one or another particular bone in the foot, then a particular muscle in the back of the knee, and so on. This approach led Carol to focus on the specifics, trying very hard to do it right. But her knees hurt.

The standard approach to pain in the knees is to work on strengthening the quadriceps muscle, but in our sessions together, we had been approaching her trouble from a different point of view: we were investigating her posture's impact on her knee. Over the past few weeks, we had looked for ways that allowed moving without effort; to play with movement instead of trying so hard; to listen, instead of commanding; to find out what could be released to allow standing, instead of working hard to stand right.

Carol began to notice how her usual posture, with her tailbone tucked under, led to tension in her hips and how that put pressure on her knees. "I think I ought to be moving my hips more when I walk. But I remember very clearly being told as a girl not to sway—how unladylike it is," Carol told me.

In response to her comment, I showed her two different styles of walking: one, pushing off from the ground, which gets the hips moving; the other, as if hanging from the sky, which leads to very little movement from side to side. "Neither one is right or good or bad," I clarified. "Hips swaying, a specific aspect of movement, is part of a certain style of moving, a whole attitude." I took a different perspective from the yoga teacher: to consider the bigger sense of moving through a space instead of moving specific body parts.

Previously, Carol and I had talked about the perils of micro-managing our movements. Our conscious minds are just not fast enough to manage the enormous number of possibilities in even the simplest gesture. Too much intention directed at the body parts can interfere with our coordination rather than improving it. "Think about moving as theatre," I say, "as play instead of parts management."

Carol went on to talk about how she felt when she was with her 11-year-old grandson—"so free, so spacious." Her eyes lit up, and her arms described a big gesture, a circle of embrace. She called it *joy*. She said, "It's such a contrast to how I feel as I go through my day. Doing my daily duties, dutifully, I feel good, but not free." As she described this state, her chest sank, her tailbone turned under, and the position of her head changed just slightly, narrowing her view. She pondered, "How did this happen! I was such a wild child, always out of doors." She said, now standing beautifully tall, "We lived on the border of 75 acres of conservation land." Gesturing gracefully with her arm, she continued, "The whole place was my estate." And there, with no effort, was the standing posture we had sought over the past weeks.

I could see each rib expand out toward the horizon, following the arm's gesture. For Carol, her standing (in both meanings of the word) changed enormously with her expansive gesture. There was a sense of legitimacy in her stance, as if she were expanding into the space surrounding her instead of shrinking from it. It was a legitimacy that didn't interfere with anyone else. Her taking up more space did not take anything away from me: on the contrary, my experience of Carol at that moment was of being welcomed by her.

The attitude expressed in Carol's phrase "The whole place was my estate" was the key to transforming her posture. She found a sense of space, giving her knees breathing room instead of compression. In contrast to the approach where we imagine the body as parts and try to control them, Carol's gesture expressed a sense of herself in relation to her surroundings. The ease in her posture emerged from an expressive process, not just a biomechanical one. Through image and language, we could touch both dimensions at once.

I call these moments of expression that can happen for a person "magic words." Like in the story of Aladdin, everyone has an "Open Sesame," words and images that open the door. Sometimes I offer some words myself, but it is most powerful when the words come directly from the person. As another client, Margaret, put it, "The words well up." Magic words are both language and movement. They come through our imagination, and they change our posture, our attitude, with no trying, no willing it, no effort. Posture, then, comes from an entirely different place from will.

Carol's story illustrates the way a gesture can have significance for an individual. It reflects an attitude, a way a person experiences their world, their environment, their options. The change in attitude allowed an important pain-free option for the biomechanics of the knee. To move with ease, the knees require that at times we find a stable connection through them and at other times we lighten their load. Carol's dutiful posture put too much consistent pressure through her knees. The change in Carol's posture when she showed "the whole place was my estate" took the pressure off the knees and allowed her to move with more ease and less pain. She could then use each option when appropriate. Physical symptoms such as Carol's knee problems are usually understood as mechanical, and the person's experience isn't considered as a factor. It's not that the symptoms are merely psychosomatic; it's that they are often a consequence of a way of meeting the environment, a way of being that relates to something in a person's experience of being in the world.

In movement practice, we start with an understanding of what standing in gravity requires, but we won't find new options by holding an effortful image of good posture. Instead, when we make space for the whole person, new options are discovered. But how do we describe "the whole person" approach? Hubert introduced us to a framework that considers four dimensions which are illustrated by Carol's story: for the knee, good biomechanics depends on good coordination between the muscles that stabilize, flex, and extend, for example. Yet for Carol, what brought about a change in the knee's coordination was a change in meaning and perception. Each of her postures reflected an attitude, a way of making meaning. They also involved different ways of perceiving the space around her. Coordination, perception, and meaning may also be considered as structures that are as important as the physical structure we see in the body's flesh. In this chapter, we are going to explore this new model of integration that Hubert shared with us that includes all four dimensions.

FOUR STRUCTURES: PHYSICAL, COORDINATIVE, PERCEPTUAL, SYMBOLIC

In 2000, after a few years' hiatus, Hubert began teaching a new group of 14 Rolfers, with a couple more experienced students like me invited as assistants. We met in the new studio Kevin Frank had built on his property in Holderness, New Hampshire, where we had held Hubert's classes for several years. From the windows, White Oak Pond glistened, and occasionally the nesting loon called to her mate.

On the first morning of the workshop, Hubert drew a simple diagram on a newsprint pad resting on an easel. It showed the four dimensions illustrated in Carol's story that Hubert called different kinds of structure:

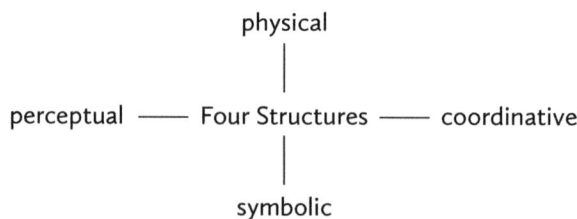

physical
|
perceptual ——— Four Structures ——— coordinative
|
symbolic

"When we want to change something, what creates the resistance?" he asked us. Usually when Rolfers think of structures related to the body, we imagine the fascia, the connective tissue and other soft tissue, bones, organs, the physical structures that make us up. As Dr. Rolf said, this is the kind of structure we can get our hands on. But it is only one of the kinds of structure that is relevant when we seek to address a symptom.

Structure and function

As moving systems, we can broaden our understanding of structure beyond the tissue scaffolding itself. Structure and function are not in opposition: they are related. Over time, function—the way we do something, move, sit, breathe, or walk—shapes our muscles and becomes our structure. As the Austrian biologist Ludwig von Bertalanffy (1901–1972) wrote, "What are called structures are slow processes of long duration, functions are quick processes of short duration" (Bertalanffy, 1952, p.134). Structure and function are two sides of the same coin, not two different domains.

Function shapes structure both in the long time span of evolution and over the shorter term of an individual's life. For example, the evolution of human bipedal gait was accompanied by changes in the shape of our ancestors' cranium and pelvis. On a personal level, we see patterns in the way each one of us learns to stand up and all the other habitual movements that make up our daily life: from sitting at school, to using phones and computers, to whether we prefer hiking or biking. All these activities shape our bodies. Norbert Weiner, cybernetics pioneer (1894–1964), wrote, "We are not stuff that abides, but patterns that perpetuate themselves" (Weiner, 1950, p.96). Habits of movement become our structure over time. The habitual way we move becomes a structure of coordination.

The structure of coordination

The concept of movements as structures, repeating patterns, was first introduced by Nikolai Bernstein (1967). Following Bernstein, researchers Tully, Turvey, and Fitch defined coordinative structure as "a functional group of muscles, often spanning many joints, that is constrained to act as a single unit" (Kelso, 1982, p.24). As we saw in Chapter Four, Hubert simplified Bernstein's research for us by explaining that we aren't giving each muscle in the body its own individual order to move. Rather, we connect all those muscles as the wheels of a car are connected by an axle. Learning a movement is creating a coordinative structure. The process reduces the degrees of freedom, so that we only have to give one command for a whole complex movement. Picture a novice learning to play tennis: at first, as the beginner moves to hit the ball, it's likely that most of the motion will be around the shoulder joint while the rest of the body will be held stiffly. But as the person builds their tennis skills, we will see more muscles involved, a more complex coordination. But the movement system is still only giving one command. Like an axle, linkages have been established. All the person needs to do is to press the start button (metaphorically) for the coordinative structure to unfold.

We won't find these connections in the tissue. They are neurological, an association that happens before moving. Just as it can be challenging to release layers of tissue that are stuck together (the "knots"), so it can be challenging to change a sequence of movements that are stuck together. The coordination pattern we have adopted may not be the most efficient, but since we are used to moving in a certain way, we just keep doing it. This is one focus of movement work: to change the coordinative structures; to open up options instead of repeating one pattern.

It's important to make a distinction between physical structure and coordinative structure, two of the four kinds of structure in Hubert's diagram. A person could have good alignment (physical structure) but still have difficulty doing the tango with ease (coordinative structure); or conversely, be a great tango dancer, while slouching around the office.

Understanding movement patterns as a kind of structure of coordination teaches us that it is a mistake to approach changing movement by trying to hold a body part in a certain way—to tuck the pelvis or hold our shoulders back. The patterned sequence of movements of coordinative structure can't be changed by muscular effort once the start button has been pushed. Instead, we will intervene in the preparation phase of movement—the pre-movement—to change the start button itself, by addressing perception.

Perception is a structure

Movement work includes changing the tissue structure, the coordinative structures, and the third kind of structure, the structures of *perception*, Hubert explained in his lecture that day in New Hampshire. Hubert described perception as a structure, a habitual pattern. "We have a way of using the perceptive organ which is a structure coming from our history," he said. "You could call it a matrix of perception." A matrix is the surrounding medium in which perception is embedded and develops. Beyond the neurological tissues and physical receptors involved, perception has its own organization. In what way can we understand perception as a structure, a repeating pattern that is stuck together?

For example, we may use our eyes in a habitual way: as we explored in Chapter Three, we might have a preference for focal vision or peripheral vision. Or one eye might specialize in surveying the periphery and the other in the details of focal vision. Each of us may also have a habit of placing the vanishing point in the visual field a certain way. The vanishing point, where parallel lines appear to converge in the distance, is a key visual cue that helps us judge distances, understand spatial relationships, and orient ourselves as we move through space. It's the way we construct spatial reality. Hubert noted that without changing the perceptive structure, we can't change body structure. "There may be a change," he said, "but it will not last too long if it isn't accompanied by a change in perspective."

Remember James Gibson's approach to perception (Chapter One): it's not the same as the passive stimulation of a sense receptor. In the context of Gibson and ecological psychology, when we talk about perception, we mean how we understand and interact with the world around us, not just what we see or hear. Perception is an activity, keeping us in touch with our surroundings, detecting useful information in the environment. What is important to pay attention to? What is meaningful? The structure of perception has to do with what information we habitually tune in to, to help us orient and take action.

Imagine walking into a room and seeing a chair. According to James Gibson's theory, the chair isn't just an object; it's something you can sit on, or stand on if you are trying to reach a high shelf. What you see are the actions the chair makes possible for you—how you can interact with it. It offers a possibility for action, which Gibson calls an "affordance" (Gibson, 1977).[1] According to Gibson, what we perceive are affordances in the environment—not neutral shapes or simple objects. Affordances are a factor that structures perception. If you are tired, then what the couch affords—a place to lie down—might get your attention more than a chair that affords upright sitting. Perception is selective, conditioned by habit. Habitually, we could look for something to collapse onto that can hold us. By recognizing and adjusting our perception of affordances, we can alter how we interact with our environment, leading to more adaptable and efficient movements, more options. With a different perception, for instance—our support from the ground or surrounding space—rather than being drawn to the couch, we might be able to detect a dance partner instead.

Perception and action

Without a change in the many choices that structure perception, it will be hard to make a long-term change in the system. Why is the perceptive structure important? Hubert said, "Because we cannot change coordination if we don't change the way we catch information." How we select information is shaped by our past preferences, by our culture, by our physical orientation to the surroundings. It is also a key part of the neurophysiology of movement, as shown by the neuroscientist Mario Wiesendanger's research on motor control (1984). The pyramidal pathway, the upper motor neurons thought to be responsible for voluntary movement, consists of about 20 million fibers that come from the motor cortex. But only a small number of these fibers go on to synapse at the spine to make the actual movement. "How many of them arrive at the spine?" Hubert asked. "Only 300,000! Ninety-eight percent of the fibers leaving the motor cortex don't go to the spine. Where do these fibers go? They go directly on to the sensory cortex, to the brain to fish for information." Wiesendanger's study challenged the oversimplified role of the motor cortex that separates "motor" from "sensory" function. Although in a dissection it is possible to separate the posterior (afferent, sensory) pathways and anterior tracts (efferent, motor) pathways, the anatomical divisions don't hold up in movement. In movement, sensory and motor work together. Wiesendanger's research tracking the pyramidal motor pathways provided a neurophysiological basis to link action and perception.

"Fishing for information"—Hubert's evocative expression—has stuck with me for so many years because it reflects a completely different way of understanding movement from the traditional emphasis on starting from the *doing*. A dancer can learn a whole choreography by studying the steps without noticing much about the feeling of moving.[2] A pianist can learn a piece of music from looking at the notes on the page. A performance can be just going through the motions, but true originality emerges from following a perceptual path. For the dancer, a subtle exhalation or sensing the ground or space around them before the movement will change the motor pattern entirely. For the pianist, learning what to listen for is perceptual training that serves their art—the quality of touch of the piano keys will change from listening for a different quality of sound. Hubert backed up this observation by describing how sensory information comes to the motor cortex from receptors all over the body and how the motor cortex accelerates one strand of information and blocks others. He described the motor cortex as making choices, in a sense, and reframed its role from simply giving orders to that of choosing information.

There are movements that accompany perception as well: perceiving and moving happen together. I hold my head or move in a certain way in order to see, or my hand moves across a surface to feel. It is common in somatic and movement traditions to say that perception is a movement, and research such as Wiesendanger's supports that perspective. As Hubert summarized, "It is the motor cortex that makes a choice of the information coming from the environment. Perception affects coordination." As in the example of seeing a chair, we see the possibility of sitting, we perceive possible actions. And actions always include how not to fall down, how to stay oriented.

As we saw in Part I, research from across academic fields supports a different paradigm from that of the objectified body split off from the environment and dominated by a bossy brain. An emphasis on changing perception to affect the way we make an action is not the standard view of exercise. Hubert summed up the difference between that view and his perspective:

> Finally, you see that the movement [the action] is completely secondary. The human being is a unity who has an exchange with the surroundings. One aspect of the exchange is movement, but the main issue is about perception, the way you select your perceptions, the way you organize the afferents [incoming signals] in your system.

Thus, it begins to make sense that when we want to change a movement, we don't start with effortful action—just doing something. Instead, we use perceptual processes to tune the coordinative structures (Kelso, 1982). As we have seen, movement begins in the preparation for action, what we have been calling pre-movement—that is also a perceptual act. The structures that shape perception are as varied as physical orientation, the timbre of the moment, or the affordances of an environment in which we find ourselves. Structures of perception and coordination are interrelated. Sometimes it is more effective to work in these domains than just trying to change the body's structure through manipulation. And there is still one more structure to consider: Hubert called the fourth structure "symbolic."

Symbolic structure

Carol's experience described at the beginning of the chapter is a good example of symbolic structure. Her dutiful posture held significance for her: it represented a mood, a weighty responsibility connected with her life as an adult, wife, and mom. This attitude changed dramatically with her gesture "the whole place was my estate." At that moment, she owned the space all around her. She stood tall and her eyes brightened as she remembered her "wild child." The posture, the mood, and the coordination of the gesture are associated with a time, a place, a memory, and an experience. They have meaning.

The term "symbol" is from *sym* which means "together" and *bol* which means "thrown." Symbolic means "thrown together." Carol's use of space and her emotional experience are tied together with her postures—the orientation to the environment and her gestures. Symbolic doesn't mean not real. While we may think of symbolic as something mental, disembodied, actually these associations have the same strength as a literal synapse. The surroundings, the emotional quality, the smells, tastes, and so on are merged in a patterned way. Our associations and interpretations, the meaning we ascribe to gesture, can also be seen as a structure. This association adds emotional context to every movement. And just like the other structures described here, there can be resistance to changing the structure of the meanings we have made.

Ten years after our first meeting, Hubert pulled together the threads of what he had been presenting for many years into the framework I have described in this chapter. Students and practitioners find it useful to this day. While presenting a theoretical framework that went beyond seeing structure as just the body's flesh, Hubert's description of the four structures was a new model of integration that had practical implications for us as Rolfers and movement teachers. Each of the four structures has plasticity: each can be an entry point for change and new possibilities. Many of us have chronic tensions that we try to change by stretching or strengthening. We don't usually think about the possibility of changing these tensions through the channel of perception, choosing different information, or through uncovering the deep symbolic associations we have established between a posture and a meaning.

This model of integration suggests that to enable a lasting change in behavior, all the dimensions of a pattern may have to be considered. This is in contrast to the usual separation—going to the Rolfer for the physical structure, to the gym or the yoga class to work on movement, and to the psychotherapist to find the meaning. Perceptual processes are often not even named as a factor. In this model, in practice, as we explored in Carol's session, integration of the four dimensions happens organically. As we approach a physical complaint through movement, we often discover underlying attitudes and gestures, beliefs, and perceptual habits, freeing ourselves for a richer exploration of embodiment. As the session with Carol shows, it is possible to include all four structures in a session: releasing restrictions in the tissue itself, looking at the coordination sequence, the pre-movement and perceptual structures, and the symbolic aspect.

Sometimes when we begin to entertain the personal significance of physical gestures, the old notion of body language comes up. Hubert often cautioned us not to assume that the shape of the body reveals the psychological profile of a person. That's an illusion, an oversimplification. The development of each person's perceptual and coordinative structures will lead to a unique combination along with the associations in each one's personal and cultural history. How do we read another person in this new model? We will explore this topic in the next chapter.

CHAPTER SEVEN

Posture Reflects Attitude

BODY READING: COMING TO MEET

At the New Hampshire workshop in the summer of 2000, we gathered together in the studio by White Oak Pond to practice "body reading" (*lecture du corps*). Years before, in the basic Rolfing training, we had practiced what Dr. Rolf and the teachers who inherited her work called "seeing." Our classmates stood in front of us, usually at a standstill, and we students tried to see a person's "organization in gravity," an important skill since a practitioner's course of action depends on it. Seeing felt like quite a challenge for a Rolfer-in-training, an opportunity to feel somewhat inadequate as we struggled to see—what exactly?

We all engage in pattern recognition without thinking too much about it. When you see your friend in the distance, you can often recognize them by their movement before you can clearly see their facial features. In a professional context, we could use tools for objective measurement. For instance, using a force platform, we could measure if our client puts the same amount of weight on each foot. Or we could do what early chiropractors did: hang a plumb line from the ceiling and have a person stand against it to see where the person's structure deviated from the line.

Body reading is different. It isn't measuring with tools, and it isn't purely intuitive either. In reading a body in motion, we are perceiving, describing, and analyzing the strategies a person uses to stay upright, how each person manages instability while in motion. This type of reading isn't done merely with the eyes. We watch someone walk, picking up an impression of the person, and then walk ourselves, allowing our own bodies to imitate what we perceive—the gestalt of the person's movement—without too much thinking. Sometimes Hubert called this unique signature a *kinetic melody* (Head, 1926, p.88).

That day, however, Hubert took a new approach. "We are going to create the theatre of coming to meet, how two people meet. The meeting is already a dramatic composition," he said. "The postural set of each person already tells us the potential of action between them. This will help you see the primary preference of how a person orients in gravity." To demonstrate, he chose Brendan, an older fellow, thin and strong, and Laney, a slender dancer.

Starting at either end of the room, Brendan and Laney walked towards each other as directed, stopping and starting several times. The rest of us stood on the sidelines, watching. Hubert asked us a few questions:

- What is the sound when they are walking?
- What is the first part that moves?
- And as they approach each other, what story is told?
- When they walk towards each other, what is the potential of action? Ready to jump? Less ready? Ready to push?

This is the theatre of potential action. If we were watching a play, what would we anticipate happening? Hubert referred to Aristotle's perspective from *Poetics* (Sachs, n.d.): the theatre is not the actors, but what happens between the actors. Even before the actors move, there is a story simmering between them. "It's one way of understanding posture," Hubert liked to say. "Posture is the potential of action." The way a person organizes themselves in gravity tells a story of possibilities. How do we read these possibilities?

Brendan had momentum in his stride, while Laney held back. His potential of action was to jump on her; hers was cautious approach, the fox crossing the ice, more care for each foot placement, testing each one before committing her weight. As Laney and Brendan walked towards each other, the potential action simmered—what would happen when they met? The theatre of meeting between Brendan and Laney revealed "body" in a new way: not as individual muscles with tension, but as a gesture that expresses something in a scene, in a relationship with another person. This body reading was not static—it wasn't simply looking at which shoulder was higher, for example, or whether the person stood straight. We were reading what our actors might be about to *do*. What we saw in each body's shape was part of a process, a sequence that had begun but was not completed. An action was suggested, prepared for, but it hadn't happened yet. Watching, we were in suspense.

POSTURE REFLECTS ATTITUDE:
PRE-MOVEMENT AND ACTION

As the participants approached each other slowly, it was clear that expression had two distinct parts: the pre-movement or preparation for action came first, separate from the behavior itself. In the space between, an emotion arose in us and between the actors. Something was communicated. Of course, Brendan did not actually jump on Laney, but his momentum opened up that possibility. What might have appeared as caution in Laney's movements would also have given her the strength and preparation to catch him if necessary!

As we meet each other in daily life, we are instinctively reading the other person. Evolution probably has prepared us to read the potential actions of others as they approach us: friendly or hostile? Ready to mate? Ready to play? In the context of theatre, the setting creates a particular situation that also affects the pre-movement and action. Our two actors might have looked different walking towards someone else, or towards a tree, or when not walking in the middle of a group of watchful colleagues! To change our movement patterns or understand another person's, we need to see the expressive gesture as a whole with the context. We allow ourselves to receive an impression from the other person, while refraining from interpretation.

To read the potential actions of Laney and Brendan included detecting the pre-movements they used to manage gravity, to not fall over while in motion. These are the pre-movements of orientation to space and to the ground—what we could call perceptual strategies. Brendan's forward momentum necessitated a sense of space; Laney's pace, a sense of the ground as support. Pre-movement for stabilization and pre-movement for action are related, since every action requires that we not fall down. No matter what we are expressing, every action begins with orienting in gravity. And the way we use gravity will offer certain possibilities: stand your ground, run away, or meet, engage, exchange.

Yet we have to be careful not to fall into making meaning beyond the potential action. We could not say what their movements meant for Brendan or Laney, but we can say how their movements affect us. You can feel yourself react if someone enters your personal space too abruptly. The most simple sense of whether we like a person or are more cautious in front of them is a form of body reading, of discerning a person's potential of action.

There are many models of somatic psychology—body-oriented psy-chology—that attribute specific meanings to certain parts of the body. For instance, in some approaches, the left side may be considered the feminine side and the right the dominant, or male. Or the brain itself has been divided into the right brain, more creative, and the left side, more intellectual. In practice, these attributions don't hold up across the board. Lived experience is much too complex to be contained in these frameworks.

Over the years of study, Hubert consistently distinguished the body reading we were engaged in from this kind of thinking, thus diverging from many systems that try to codify or make a lexicon of meaning of each muscle. "Each part of the body does not have a meaning in itself. It has a function based on how I have constructed my gestures, based on how I have built the narrative of my life" (Montreux workshop, 2009). We can't read the psychological underpinnings of a person from the shape of their body. Each human experience leads to a particular way of organizing ourselves that has meaning to us, through us. The meanings emerge from a particular person's history and culture and in a particular context. For each person, the associations will be a different story, a different meaning.

It is so important not to impose our own interpretation on another's gesture. Frankly, it's easier to ask, to inquire, to find out from the person in question what that person's experience might be. We can create the-atre opportunities for ourselves, taking on different starting points and noticing the impact on ourselves and the other person. It's remarkable to realize that behind many aspects of expressive life are small choices of perceptual strategy. As we will see, it's at that level that we can impact them in ourselves and others.

POSTURE REFLECTS AN ATTITUDE

As Hubert's theatre scene revealed that day, a person's posture expresses something more than mechanics. As Laney and Brendan walked towards each other, we could see the possibilities that emerged from their interac-tion and begin to discern the perceptual strategies underlying the poten-tial of action; the information they were selecting and the behaviors that selection made possible.

Posture reflects an attitude. Hubert has used this expression for years. What does he mean? How do we read the attitude behind posture? We have to come back to our orientation in gravity. That's what shapes our potential for action as we saw with Laney and Brendan—before any action. This organization always *precedes* the action—the system adjusts ahead of time in anticipation of changes in the center of gravity.

Pre-movement, the anticipatory activity in preparation for a movement, has both a practical, mechanical dimension and an expressive dimension.

Imagine someone extending their arm towards you, starting with a flexed arm and then extending it towards you with the palm facing up and open. We would describe this movement as flexion and extension of the forearm. Depending on the situation, the gesture could be that of royalty showing you their favor, or the very same flexion and extension could be a panhandler asking for a dollar. The meaning of the gesture is not conveyed just in the movement of the arm. Of course, the theatre scene, the context, also contributes clues to the meaning of gesture. But Hubert was pointing out something more subtle when he said, "What changes the meaning of my arm is the postural activity behind it."

A given body part in itself does not have one meaning across different contexts and neither do gestures. In Hubert's words, "You can't make a dictionary of movement. You can't say that movement is a language in which each gesture can be defined." For example, crossed arms don't automatically signify a defensive posture, but could imply a multitude of circumstances: the person might feel cold, and the arms are crossed for warmth, or perhaps they have an injury and are using their arms to help support their upright posture. The gesture in itself does not reveal the meaning.

In his talk that day, Hubert was pointing out that the meaning of the gesture comes from the pre-movement. If I raise my hand in a stop gesture, depending on how I have organized the pre-movement, it can be an expression of fear or strength. There is a pre-movement that activates a powerful stabilizer chain from the ground through the deeper trunk muscles, with serratus anterior stabilizing the shoulder blade—a powerful "Stop!" Or, if the pre-movement is a fearful contraction with pectoralis minor working first, for example, then this source of strength is not accessible, and the scapula ends up unsupported, weakening the strength of the arms. The die is cast before the arm is even raised.

As in the theory of gestalt perceptual psychology, in the figure/ground framework it is the background that gives the meaning to the gesture, not the movement itself. The social and physical contexts are part of the background, but a less commonly perceived element is the person's pre-movement. Hubert continued:

> What changes the meaning? It is the postural activity, and not the movement. This is huge: the pre-movement, what I call tonic function, in fact, is absolutely important. To be clear about it, this pre-movement, this postural anticipatory activity, is just about gravity.

In this sense, the anticipatory activity, the pre-movement discussed in Chapter Two, shapes the meaning conveyed by a gesture. As we saw in the scene with Brendan and Laney earlier in this chapter and in Carol's session in Chapter Six, the pre-movements of orientation or perceptual selection that stabilize us are also part of an expressive gesture—they prepare an action and communicate an attitude both to ourselves and to another person. The pre-movements show something about how a person experiences the world.

An attitude is not just an idea or a mental event: it is a motor pattern, a particular combination of muscular contractions that becomes a posture. In ecological psychology, a posture is an animal's orientation in relation to the environment (Reed, 1982, p.118). That orientation makes certain actions possible; it prepares us for an action that has not been completed.

Nina Bull, another somatic pioneer, also recognized the importance of pre-movement and connected it with emotion. In *The Attitude Theory of Emotion* (1951/1968), she describes attitude as "mediating the mind/body relationship" (p.xvi). Her hypothesis was that an emotion results from a pre-movement that is not expressed in an action. Being on the verge of tears is a pre-movement involving neuromuscular activity. If we don't actually burst into tears, if we inhibit the action, that is when the feeling of sadness arises. She postulated that the perceived emotion comes after the motor preparation, the pre-movement. When the action—the tears in this example—doesn't occur, then the feeling of sadness colors our world. The term "attitude" carries both meanings: a physical attitude or posture and an emotional attitude, a way of meeting the world. Attitude is an expression we pick up on in body reading.

For each of us, some of these attitudes have been practiced so often that they accompany us all the time. They become our style, what we sometimes call personality. Hubert called this the *pré-mouvement du matin*, the morning pre-movement we put on as we get out of bed. These pre-movements, this attitude, also influence our other actions. In the example of Carol from Chapter Six, she could put on her dutiful attitude at times, slightly sinking under the weight of responsibilities. The physical tensions that create Carol's dutiful posture shape her next action. How can she fully reach up in her yoga pose if, before she even begins, she is experiencing the drag of her responsibilities?

Our postures and attitudes are interwoven with how we organize our stability in gravity. For Hubert and Dr. Rolf, rather than work with the story, the emotional content and memories, through conversation, we could directly address the gestalt of human experience by working with our orientation in gravity. It is from this vantage point that we can access new options directly.

EMBODIMENT: THE CHARACTER KNOT

Hubert came up with a term "the character knot" to help us see the pattern of contraction that precedes almost any other action. You can try this for yourself. Using the example of the *stop* gesture described above, we can practice finding strength instead of contraction.

With a physioball at about shoulder height, press the ball against a wall to feel your baseline "push." Feel where your body tightens and compresses.

Try a few times, starting over each time, letting yourself detect the tiny movement that *precedes* the action, even before you push; perhaps just before you even begin to raise your arm—that's your character knot. For example, you may be able to notice a tiny compression, a gathering in, or a little tension around the tailbone or a tiny change in the orientation of your head.

Try with the other hand, to see if the pattern of contraction is the same or different.

Going back to the first side again, instead of thinking "push," let yourself notice the quality of contact of your hand with the ball and of your feet with the floor. Soften the contact with the floor. Soften your gaze. How does that change the feeling in your hand?

Next, instead of only paying attention to the space between your body and the wall, imagine the back half of your body expanding into the space behind and all around you. How does that change your sense of pushing?

In this example, accessing the ground and the space behind you are ways of changing your orientation in gravity that allow you to find a different coordination and perhaps to experience a different kind of strength—to untie the "character knot."

THE FENCING BEAR

Years before, Hubert introduced us to a story by Heinrich von Kleist to illustrate his point about gravity organization and body reading. In the story, a nobleman—an expert fencer—visited a friend at his castle. Challenged to a fencing match by the host's eldest son, the nobleman easily bested him. "You may have beaten me, but I know an opponent against whom you will not triumph!" the son said, leading him out into the yard. There, to the nobleman's surprise, stood a bear chained to a stake.

The son urged the nobleman to engage the bear in a fencing match. Each time the fencer tried to touch the bear with his rapier, the bear easily parried the thrust. But when the fencer used his most skillful feints that would have fooled any other opponent, the bear did not react at all.

Kleist's bear was an expert body reader, paying attention to where the nobleman's weight rested. The bear was never distracted by the nobleman's attempts to fake a sword thrust. He sensed that the fencer's weight was not committed and did not react. Only when there was an actual shift in his opponent's center of gravity was the bear provoked to action. This is the same skill used by successful basketball players. As practitioners, this is an important part of what we learn to read: we watch where the weight rests and how it shifts.

Kleist's 1810 "On the Marionette Theatre," in which the story of the fencing bear appears, is a four-part tale.[1] It begins with the narrator discovering the lead dancer of the Opera watching a puppet show in a marketplace in Berlin. The narrator expresses some surprise that the puppets would appeal to such a skilled dancer. But Herr C., the dancer in question, describes the grace he finds in the puppets' movements. He explains to the puzzled narrator that each of a puppet's limbs does not need to be controlled independently; instead, the movement itself has a center of gravity. All the puppet master has to do is manage that one point and the limbs will follow. I remember my delight at the time to read a story from so long ago in which the power of gravity featured so prominently.

In addition, the dancer explains, the puppets have a big advantage in having no self-consciousness. They are, like our robots from Chapter

Two, entirely free of body image—how I imagine I appear to you, the Other—that can get in the way of the grace of our human movements.

Kleist's character states: "Affectation appears, as you know, when the soul, *vis motrix*, inhabits any other point than the center of gravity."[2] Again the story echoed what we were learning in body reading: what seems like a primarily physical or mechanical phenomenon of how weight or load is managed also impacts the feeling we pick up from another person. Authentically grounded or just a faker?

The puppets have another advantage: they have strings to lift them, and only have to graze the ground to benefit from a little counterforce, whereas humans inevitably need the ground to rest and recover. Kleist's story raised a question that we had been puzzling over since first meeting Hubert: he described *two* directions that gravity's signals give us—orientation to ground and to space. How we use these two information sources is a fundamental aspect of movement that we will explore in the next chapter.

CHAPTER EIGHT

Patterns of Orientation

It's 1995. In the summer house by White Oak Pond, we watch a video of Fred Astaire and Gene Kelly dancing together in a skit from the Ziegfeld Follies, "The Babbitt and the Bromide" (Warner Bros. Classics, 2016). Although the two dancers had performed together in many films, it was rare to see them dancing identical choreography, side by side.

Frame by frame, Hubert pointed out Gene Kelly's muscular approach in contrast to Astaire's airier feel. Astaire's jumps took him more aloft, a little higher each time than Kelly. Astaire embodied lightness with a sense of space and grace, as if he were suspended by invisible puppet strings. Kelly seemed to draw power from connecting to the ground. There was a sense of strength and weight about him, compared to Astaire's airy style.

Hubert used the video to show the students in the workshop how the two dancers used different styles of orientation to begin their movements. These styles could also be described as two different ways of sensing weight. Although we don't often stop to think about it, weight represents the force exerted on us by earth's gravitational field. It's an ongoing acceleration, a force with a direction, not a static event. We can sense this linear acceleration through our inner ear and vestibular system. We can also sense the ground pushing up against us through the proprioceptors in our joints and muscles. Each dancer subconsciously chose one of these frames of reference, signals, or sources of information to start with, to help him organize his balance while dancing beautifully (Berthoz, 1997/2000). Hubert explained that while we have multiple sensors that can convey gravity's signals to our brains in the course of a movement, we often have a preference of starting point: Astaire's sense of weight came *first* through vestibular information, while Kelly's sense of weight came *irst* through sense receptors embedded in the soles of the feet.

Hubert gave us another example of contrasting choices of orientation in sports: Olympic track-and-field athletes Ben Johnson and Carl Lewis. Ben Johnson seemed to pull the ground, giving him explosive power; while Carl Lewis' capacity for spatial orientation was apparent in the orientation of his head, his lofty stance (NHL Overtimes, 2021). Each athlete maintained his orientation by tuning into gravity as a source of information—even before he moved—but they did so using different primary sources of information.

As discussed earlier, actions are always preceded by movements that anticipate and prepare for the effects on our balance. Orienting is the first pre-movement, a necessary element preceding all other movements. We need to be oriented to keep from falling when we go into motion, and we need it just to stand up. It is part of the set-up that is required for a sequence of movements, such as throwing a ball, or walking, or using our keyboards at the computer. Even the most basic actions, like looking at something or breathing, begin with an orientation to gravity. Orienting is the movement we repeat the most often, but because it is *pre*-movement that comes before any visible sign of action, its importance often goes unrecognized. The falling robots described in Chapter Two are an example of this: the engineers missed something essential for movement. All animals have to have a way of orienting in gravity in order to keep from falling over while moving.

Here in a terrestrial environment, being oriented in gravity depends on being able to sense which way is up and which way is down. As Gibson describes it:

> [T]he simplest kind of orientation [is] to the direction up-down and to the plane of the ground. Along with this goes a basic type of perception on which other perceptions depend, that is, the detection of the stable permanent framework of the environment. This is sometimes called the perception of "space," but that term implies something abstract and intellectual, whereas what is meant is something concrete and primitive—a dim, underlying, and ceaseless awareness of what is permanent in the world. (Gibson, 1966, p.59)

Non-consciously, we select certain cues from the environment for orientation. Usually, we think about one center of gravity, but in the passage quoted above, Gibson describes two categories—ground and space. Hubert suggested that each one of us initiates our gestures primarily from one or the other. The initial choice affects the rest of the sequence of action for every movement. Astaire's orientation suggested that he started with a sense of space—every movement began with reaching up or out—which goes together with tuning more to the information from his inner ear and to the surrounding space. Kelly's preference of orientation was to the ground: he connected with the seat or the floor before moving, primarily tuning into information coming through the proprioceptors in the muscles and joints and the pressure receptors in the soles of the feet that give us a sense of where we are.

The examples of famous dancers and athletes show us in broad strokes the effects of using different strategies of orientation, how our preference of orienting strategy shapes us physically. As the movement we do the most often, our pre-movement strategy determines which muscles will get recruited for action. Kelly and Johnson pushed off the ground, leading to a more (phasic) muscular frame; the floating style of Astaire and Lewis kept their muscles long and lithe (mostly tonic muscles). The basic pattern of orientation influences how we move and eventually shows up in the actual physical shape of each one's body, as well as in each of his steps. That is true for all of us.

Regardless of their differences, Gene Kelly and Fred Astaire were both fabulous dancers, and Lewis and Johnson accomplished athletes. Although each one of us may have an aesthetic preference or unconscious bias for one style over the other, neither orientation is right or wrong. Like all of us, the dancers and athletes are using multiple sources of information—vestibular and proprioceptive as well as visual—to stay upright and move in the gravitational field. They are just exhibiting a preference for initiating movement with one over the other.

Different actions are made available depending on the pre-movement or the style of orientation. For Ben Johnson, the explosive capacity of phasic muscle showed up at the very start of the race and for the first 50 meters, while the long-duration capacity of tonic muscles gave Lewis the advantage in the second half of a race. For pulling and pushing, we need a good ground orientation. To prepare for sliding, gliding, and jumping, space orientation might provide more useful information to organize the movement initially.

We can read another's potential of action; we can also perceive orientation strategies. We can't "read" an interpretation of the meaning these choices hold for each individual, although it is important to recognize that there can be an attitude or emotional association behind the preferences we express and the ones we avoid.

PERCEPTUAL SYSTEMS AND ORIENTATION

Hubert's experience in dance and teaching movement echoed Gibson's perspective: perception does not describe a flow of passively incoming sensations. Instead, it is picking up on the important information the environment provides, information about orientation (Gibson, 1966). In everyday discourse, the terms "sensation" and "perception" may be equated; however, this casual use hides a very important distinction, almost a difference in worldview. Are animals just passively receiving sensations that inherently "make sense"? Or are we actively selecting— choosing—information from our environment?

Gibson's perspective is once again useful: he thought of the senses as active, exploratory, and interrelated systems, which he called perceptual systems:

> We shall have to conceive the external senses in a new way, as active rather than passive, as systems rather than channels, and as inter-related rather than mutually exclusive. If they function to pick up information, not simply to arouse sensations, this function should be denoted by a different term. They will here be called perceptual systems. (Gibson, 1966, p.47)

Gibson suggested that this shift from a classical view of the senses as passive to thinking of perceptual systems opens the door to skill building. Each of our receptors is sensitive to a certain kind of input—that is a given. But perceptual systems are all about learning. With practice, we can improve our capacity to orient in different situations, for different actions. We can tune our listening, refine our sense of touch, and bring increased clarity to our visual capacity.

Taking Gibson's point of view of perceptual systems lets us see ourselves in a new light: the body is not an object; it is an *activity*. Embodiment, living as a body, requires ongoing choices of perceptual information. Our perceptual choices affect how we orient, how we prepare to move, and the subsequent mechanics of our actions. A slightly different use of gaze, a slightly different sense of space, a slightly different way of contacting the ground through the feet, all result in a different pattern of muscular recruitment that in turn leads to a difference in body shape.

Daily, unconsciously, we are shaping ourselves through our perceptual and movement preferences, creating the shape of our bodies over time. Yet exercise and the traditional approach to rehabilitation tend to keep the focus on individual muscles or muscle groups, strength building, and reps. The underlying pre-movements and perceptual skills aren't part of the practice. Although it is now possible to show that each person has a unique movement signature, the research has yet to suggest what leads to it, and how our movement habits can get us into trouble. What more do we need to understand about pre-movements to use this important information? How do these unconscious pre-movements help or hinder us in action?

Our habits of perception are directly connected to how we organize ourselves in response to the force of gravity. In Gibson's terminology, the orienting system is part of every perception and action. Without realizing it, we must manage our orientation even just to look at something. Because of this intimate relationship between managing uprightness and the perceptual information we pick up from our surroundings, we can't change our perceptual habits without including orientation. Our orientation in gravity is already shaping what we perceive; it is shaping our potential for action. Remember, this organization always *precedes* the action—the system adjusts ahead of time for changes in the center of gravity. What is the impact on us of these unconscious choices? How do we influence them to affect orientation, perception, and action?

ORIENTING AND STABILIZING

"You can't saw off the branch you are sitting on," Hubert said one day during a rare workshop series for French speakers in the Rolfing community. It was 2008, and we were high in the Alps in the mountain town of Chandolin, in Switzerland. He said it light-heartedly, but the saying has stuck with me for years. He meant that whatever perceptual strategy you use for stabilizing—a pre-movement that serves orientation—leads to a pattern of use in which some muscles get more work and others rarely get recruited. You use a particular series of muscular contractions to stabilize yourself, which means that you are loading that area, putting your weight on it. That's the "branch you are sitting on" in Hubert's metaphor. You can't stop using that source of support without first finding a different one.

Let's say a person seeks help with a shoulder problem. In the usual thinking for rehabilitation, a practitioner would try to correct the movement restriction at the shoulder by releasing the tissue and/or by strengthening the muscles around the shoulder joint itself—for example, in the arms or chest. But, of course, as Dr. Rolf wrote, "In a balanced body, when flexors flex, extensors extend" (Rolf, 1977, p.65). In other words, the extensors have to let go to allow the movement. The letting go is as important as the action, and its quality, timing, et cetera color the movement. That means that tension that pulls down on the chest will interfere with the range of free movement at the shoulder joint. In this example, Hubert's approach would have us start by exploring what would allow the tension pulling down on the chest to let go. That would help release the shoulder so it could function properly. The orientation pattern, the choice of how to stabilize, comes first.

If you are using that particular strategy to keep from falling over, then the muscles involved won't be able to let go to participate in the delicate orchestration that movement requires. When a muscle is not free to let go at the appropriate time and to the degree required by a given action because it is involved in a stabilizing activity, this tension interferes with movement at the related joints (Nashner & Cordo, 1981).

Any pattern or unconscious preference of orientation in gravity that is expressed too frequently is likely to provoke a symptom eventually. The pattern of use will create or contribute to tension and overuse of certain muscles, which is often the basis of chronic pain. Unlike a worldview in which there is one right way, understanding orientation as part of every movement automatically points at our need for more than one strategy to manage changing circumstances.

We don't know where our habitual patterns of orientation originate—whether they are innate or acquired. But once recognized, we can work with our habit of orientation; we can practice "re-sourcing" our pre-movement. For example, we can develop such strong invisible marionette strings that we rest all the way into the ground like Fred Astaire, or we can learn to go from the ground to find the sky like Gene Kelly. Learning to vary the sources of perceptual information gives us adaptability, which is a sustainable long-term strategy for movement. That is the skill we can cultivate.

VESTIBULAR SYSTEM AND SENSE OF SELF

Vestibular information, the primary source for Astaire's style, is essential for movement and balance, but not as widely recognized as such in popular culture. When people say "I need to get more grounded," most of them are thinking about feeling the earth, feeling their feet on the ground. But the information our inner ears are picking up on is also a way of sensing weight, of being well oriented, and is crucial to knowing where we are in space.

Hubert mentioned research exploring the unusual capacity of African women from Kikiyu and Luo tribes who carry heavy pots of water on their heads. The research showed that the women's movements were actually *more* efficient in terms of oxygen consumption rate when they were carrying the heavy weight than when they were just walking. In addition, the women actually accomplished a *better* transfer of energy in the pendulum-like movement of walking when carrying a load (Heglund *et al.*, 1995). The research did not specify the mechanism that led to the increase in conservation of energy for the African women. Hubert's conjecture was that if the information—the pressure from the pot—had to travel all the way to the ground before there was a response to the effects on the woman's center of gravity, it would take too long to coordinate balancing the heavy pot while walking. The increased information to the otoliths—the crystals in the inner ear that detect gravity—may be what helped the movement organize even better than without the extra weight of the pot, thus supporting the idea that human beings have two ways to sense gravity.

The vestibular system's function, however, goes far beyond efficiency. In *The Brain that Changes Itself* (2007), Canadian psychiatrist Norman Doidge writes vividly about a patient with severe damage to her inner ear. A woman in her 40s, Cheryl felt that she was falling, continuously. Even when she actually did fall to the floor, the sensation remained. She could only walk with difficulty, feet wide apart and leaning on a cane. As movement was so challenging and the falling feeling was ever present, she couldn't work and experienced enormous anxiety. Balance—another of the senses, though not included in Aristotle's original list—is impossible without accurate information to the brain's vestibular cortex. When something went wrong, Doidge writes, it affected all aspects of Cheryl's being.

Cheryl's story had a happy ending. Paul Bach-y-Rita, an ingenious neuroscientist, invented a device that allowed signals given to her tongue to replace the missing input from the inner ear, providing a different stream of information for her brain's vestibular nuclei to use. The invention worked far better than researchers had imagined: in addition to providing the immediate sensory substitution, it enabled a kind of training for Cheryl's brain such that eventually she hardly needed to use the device at all.

Cheryl's success beautifully proves Gibson's point: the senses are perceptual systems that can be trained. Without that understanding, Bach-y-Rita might never have undertaken his valuable experiment. Like Fred Astaire and Gene Kelly, Cheryl had been tuning in to one stream of information to organize her balance, but with the help of Bach-y-Rita's invention, she was able to learn to tune in to a different information source. That is also an example of neuroplasticity, the point of view that describes how our brains function, that came to light during the second half of the 20th century.

Regardless of how we go about getting them, messages about which way is up are essential for moving and are deeply tied to a secure sense of self. Alain Berthoz,[1] a neurophysiologist who specializes in multisensory integration and the brain's sense of movement, classified the vestibular system as "*the basic frame of reference* of all our perception of space and for constructing our sense of our bodies vis-à-vis the world" (Berthoz, 2009, p.148; my italics and translation). Berthoz asserts that the vestibular system contributes to our (and other animals') ability to combine information from our different senses into a coherent worldview. For human beings, how we manage gravity is not merely a mechanical problem, but an aspect of our sense of self.

PATTERNS OF ORIENTATION AND METAPHOR

While we can use the simplicity of the concepts of ground and space to orient our own thinking or pattern recognition as we did when we compared Fred Astaire's and Gene Kelly's styles, it would be an oversimplification to turn the concepts into a fixed typology, to label ourselves as "up" or "down" types. In practice, each functional part of the body— foot, shoulder, chest—could have more of a ground orientation, a sense of weight resting, or more of a space orientation, lightness at any given moment. To push a heavy dresser, we need the strength that comes from the ground. We need adaptability—to increase one direction (ground) without losing the other (sky). What is important are the *two* directions, the polarity—in fact, we need them both, and their ongoing relationship is one of the most foundational of human experiences. As such, the theme appears in many contexts.

During a visit with Hubert in 2006, Hubert pointed out the complex interplay of the two directions in his analysis of the famous painting by Raphael, "The School of Athens." [Figure 7]

Figure 7: "The School of Athens"

In the detail depicted in Figure 8, we see Plato, gesturing upwards, and Aristotle, with his palm pointing down. The gesture of each of the two central figures reflects their respective philosophical positions, Plato seeking archetypal forms beyond appearances, and Aristotle grounded in the categories of the material world. But at the same time, their gestures *oppose* their overall orientation as depicted by the artist. We see/feel the weight represented in Plato's head and chest, and even in the heavy folds of his earth-colored robe, while Aristotle's head and neck soar along with the sky-blue fabric that seems to float around him. Part of the beauty and mystery of the painting is the interplay of this polarity. [Figure 8]

I was reminded of Gaston Bachelard, the French philosopher who wrote, "of all metaphors, metaphors of height, elevation, depth, sinking, and the fall are the axiomatic metaphors par excellence" (Bachelard *et al.*, 2011, p.10). We are all intimately familiar with the sensations evoked by such imagery. Descriptions of the two directions convey an immediate felt experience to almost any reader.

Bachelard points out that the vertical axis also has a moral dimension: along with poets and thinkers like Shelley and Nietzsche, he attributes positive value to lightness and upward movement, and a negative sense to "the fall." In contrast, in the contemporary thought of James Hillman (2021), the same vertical axis is described as the tension between spirit, which always seeks the heights and open spaces, and soul, which stays low in the depths and valleys. In Hillman's version of morality, we have neglected the importance of the depths in favor of the heights. He calls the relationship between spirit and soul a difficult marriage with no possibility of divorce. Regardless of which direction carries which value, both authors recognize a psychological dimension in experiences of heavy/light, down/up.

Figure 8: Detail of "The School of Athens"

My own many years of practice support this: I have found that people relate immediately in a practical, usable way to orienting with a sense of two directions. In addition to the direct *physical* impact, there is almost always a psychological dimension, but one that is quite personal. Space can be spacious or spacey; ground can be sensed as a place of solid support, a heavy, stuck place, or even an experience of death. These metaphors take on importance for us because they are a felt experience. The gravity of our planet gives us a sense of weight.

The importance of these metaphors in our experiential world is a reflection of the context in which life takes place. Our primary relationship is with gravity: we are constantly adjusting, dynamic, actively orienting in the field of gravity. The gravitational pull can be experienced as tension or as support depending on how we relate to it.

As we have seen throughout this book, in spite of the common cultural tendency to put cognition first, neurologists and philosophers suggest that it is actually the body's movement that shapes thinking, as much as the other way around (Jostmann *et al.*, 2009; Lakoff, 2012; Llinás, 2002). From our first moment of breath, there is a sense of weight; we learn about support in the arms of our nurturers. Later, as we stand up and walk, we discover a new relationship with gravity, along with a new autonomy from our caregivers. Our bodies are equipped with their own gravity-sensing system, which we call the tonic system, because the basic tone of all the muscles is a function of the relationship between the same two directions of orientation: resting and reaching, ground and space. The personal sense of two directions and its ubiquity in art and philosophy are rooted in a foundational experience of the world: a physical body in a relationship with the force of gravity.

EMBODIMENT: EXPLORING G'

The metaphorical and the practical go hand in hand. In this embodiment practice, we can explore how the perceptual preferences that we have been describing express themselves in walking.

Hubert introduced us to the work of Raymond Sohier, a contemporary Belgian physical therapist. Sohier described two walking styles: one that begins from above and the other from below (Sohier & Haye, 1989). Sohier's categories echoed Hubert's observations, with a significant difference. Rather than focusing on typing people as *from above* or *from below*, Hubert emphasized the perceptual strategy which we could use as a helpful tool to open up options in our own or our client's movement patterns.

Remember the idea of G' from the Introduction: a secondary, or partial, center of gravity—the center of gravity of the chest, arms, and head, located approximately in front of the fourth thoracic vertebra (T4). G' can be seen in motion in reference to an imaginary line running between heads of the two femurs (the trans-coxo-femoral (TCF) axis). As the movement of taking a step is initiated, G' can move in front of or behind the TCF axis. If there is a coordinative preference—always moving behind, for instance—this tends to accompany a ground orientation or walking from below. When the first step is initiated by moving G' forward of the TCF axis, that tends to go with space orientation or walking from above. Now we can understand the practices mentioned in the Introduction to change G', as well as this embodiment practice, as approaches to help open possibilities of orientation—managing our relationship with gravity—using the tools of perception we have been exploring.

What's significant about G'? Instead of seeing ourselves like a structure that is built from the ground up, we take a developmental point of view. A baby is already organizing their head movements to keep their eyes level, and their arm movements to reach for objects and people, long before even being able to sit independently, let alone stand.[2] The movement patterns of the upper body, arms, and head are organized through reaching while lying down and eventually from a sitting position. The responsiveness of that balancing act (how G' moves in relation to the TCF in sitting) will shape how center of gravity ends up over the reference line provided by Chopart's joint in the feet.

To address the responsiveness of G', we might start in sitting, letting G' slide forward and back a little bit between the shoulder blades, with the hips stationary.

Then letting the hips roll forward and back in relation to G'—letting G' momentarily act as a fixed point of reference.

As a dynamic system, different coordinations and different perceptions become available as we explore taking different starting points or priming the movement in different ways.

We can explore standing up, getting over our feet, while allowing G' to stay back a little, softening the spine's extension, standing up like a warrior, and returning to sit.

Then, allow G' to move forward first as we stand up, opening out to the world. These are only two examples of different associations we might bring to these different movement patterns. What are yours?

EMBODIMENT: SUN SALUTE

Movement practices tend to be handed down as forms: whether it is ballet instructions, Joe Pilates' syllabus, yoga asanas, or tai chi forms, the movement disciplines are often identified through their exercises. But too often, the focus is on trying to replicate the shape of the movement. The practices can become performances, repeated from memory, like the ballet dancer who practiced in front of the mirror for hours and now is performing in front of an audience, a new mirror. The problem? The movement has lost its aliveness. Hubert sometimes said a dancer could have "too much body," and that imagining how you look to someone else while moving was "the end of movement."

Hubert's framework gave me a way to grasp that movement forms could be enlisted in the service of changing my attitude instead of repeating it. Instead of being defined by a series of poses, all forms of movement became an expression of an understanding of what goes into moving in the world: pre-movement and patterns of orientation in the gravitational field lie beneath all movements and gestures. Working with our own patterns of orientation offered an approach that could be applied across many movement traditions.

What Hubert called "the sun salute" provides a good example.

Over many years of yoga classes, I had been exposed to the linked series of poses called Sun Salutation. There were variations from class to class, but they were all recognizable—the poses led from one to the next: standing, forward bend, Downward Dog pose into Warrior pose, et cetera. From the beginning of studying with Hubert, we used the Sun Salutation as a movement practice in workshops, but each time, he brought in a different point of view, a different starting point or attitude.

Version 1: An infinite line in two directions

The first time, Hubert directed us to keep a sense of a center line, imagining the line going out in two directions, extending up to the sky (or out to the surrounding space) and down through the earth. We were directed not to worry about form or shape, but instead to allow a spacious feeling to continue throughout the movement. All we were attending to was the basics of being well organized in gravity, ground, and sky. Surprisingly, without a deliberate focus on breathing, each movement brought inhaling or exhaling, without effort. The movement itself became the breath, filling, emptying, pausing, and filling again with the next gesture.

Try it for yourself. Imagine a line going out in two directions extending up to the sky (or out to the surrounding space) and down through the earth, as you move through the movements of your version of the Sun Salutation, or you could just walk slowly, letting yourself feel the earth and the space around you each step, one breath per step. Some people respond better to imagining the infinite line coming towards them from sky and ground. What works best for you to access your sense of ground and your sense of space?

Version 2: Greeting the sun

Another time, Hubert pointed out that all movements in the sun salutation are just that: a salute, a welcoming. For me, saying hello to the sun completely changed the feeling: the movement begins with a happy recognition, a gaze that in itself sets up the movement of the arms. Instead of lifting my arms, I had a sense of reaching and receiving. Again, Hubert's invitation kept us out of our doing-and-efforting attitudes and allowed an experience of the movement as a meeting, an inquiry. This approach was very different from performing the poses as I remembered them, or how I thought they should look. Following the Sun Salutation movements as Hubert instructed was also different from following a yoga teacher's movements, imitating what we saw before us. I had done the poses and worked with breath, but I never imagined how much starting to move in relationship with the sun could change the way the movement felt. It opened it up. It changed my focus from my-body-doing-this to a sense of relationship as the basis for moving. There was room for the unknown, a movement renewed each time instead of practiced.

This attitude, of welcoming or greeting, can be practiced any time. Simply raise your arms, the way you do in so many exercise routines. Then change the initiation so that before you raise your arms, you conjure up the sky or the sun as a friend or just imagine someone you love in front of you. What is the gesture you make to welcome them? We still see the arms in motion, but the whole system has changed.

Version 3: Flight of the eagle

In another workshop, Hubert had us do a series of movements he called "Flight of the Eagle." Technically, Flight of the Eagle could be described as a modified version of the Sun Salutation, but rather than having the hands on the floor, we used a chair and followed a sequence of movements that resembled the familiar one. But Hubert was asking for something different from us than anything I had experienced in a yoga class. Over several years, he put together this sequence to avoid the difficulties beginners often experience in the Sun Salutation. With too much challenge, the pre-movements—the most important part of the movement!—will be eclipsed by contraction and effort. The movements in Flight of the Eagle were carefully organized to allow each of us to pay attention to the important pre-movements in each part of the sequence instead of being hampered by any lack of flexibility.

A. Hands and feet: Letting the body disappear

Hubert's initial instructions were to forget about everything but where the hands touch the chair and the feet touch the floor. We were to feel the whole movement as the weight transferred between chair and floor, and back again—from the floor through the heel of the foot to the heel of the hand, the midfoot to the palm, the toes to the fingers and back again, in touch with the surfaces, the chair and floor. I wasn't to try to place my sacrum right, or get myself to lengthen, or give myself any kind of command. With this approach, in a surprising paradox, the body could "disappear" while being fully present, liberated by the attention to the meeting of hands and chair, feet and floor. The movements weren't about stretching hamstrings, back, or arms. They weren't about getting the pose right or imitating someone else's form. They were about practicing a different way of being in the world, being in touch. As with the *Stick work* (Introduction), this quality of contact through the hands and feet wakes up core activity, which will facilitate the rest of the movements that follow.

Although the changes we were attending to might seem based in imagination, I felt the biomechanical effects from this indirect approach. I know from experience with myself and my clients that if we practice greeting the sun every day, we get a strong core, but if we try to get a strong core directly (for instance, with repeated abdominal crunches), we often end up hurting our backs.

B. Being a warrior

In the movements that are known as Warrior 1, instead of thinking of the shape of the pose—a lunge with arms raised—the focus would be on guiding our perception to allow the weight to rest through the forward leg, so we could feel the foot receiving the floor—choosing to prioritize finding stability through sensing rather than focusing on the look of the movement. Hubert would remind us, "You are educating the cerebellum, teaching the cerebellum to find the good information." The movement's purpose isn't to "lift the arms and do a lunge" or to develop muscle strength or even flexibility, but to change the whole system. That is exactly what we are practicing: an embodiment of this ongoing relationship—brain, body, and environment—through gaze, through touch, through imagining.

C. Inventing the space

In another part of Flight of the Eagle, with our hands and feet as before, Hubert suggested we use our imagination to invent the space that surrounded us. "Imagine you are invited into the space beyond your head, and beyond your tailbone," he said. Or we could "wait to be asked," as in the practice we had done in our very first workshop, waiting for a call from the space beyond the head, beyond the tailbone. The more we did movements this way, the less the body was the focus. The focus shifted from inside the body or from the image of the body (i.e., the image of the spine articulating each vertebral segment) to a relationship with the surrounding space, a sense of actions possible in the space—going beyond our own flesh.

Beyond the mechanics, moving depends on perceptual processes. What we choose to pay attention to, how we put our world together, that's our attitude. It's a choice, a selection. There isn't one simple reality available for us to perceive. Perception is an action—something we construct—and movement depends on perception. Hubert would use evocative phrases: "Proprioception is 50 percent body, 50 percent world," "Perception is an acceleration," "Perception is selective" (Berthoz, 1997/2000, p.88), "Perception is imagination," or he would invite us to "construct the space." He would encourage us in each moment to encounter the world open to a different pre-movement, to invite something new.

Thus far, we have considered several dimensions of pre-movement: a pre-movement of orientation, a pre-movement of attitude, and a pre-movement of action and context. There is yet another important dimension: pre-movements sometimes reveal the movements or feelings we habitually avoid. We will explore this in the next chapter.

CHAPTER NINE

The Missing Gesture

CLIENT STORY: RHEA

Rhea was a cellist who came to me by referral from another musician. Five years earlier, while riding her bike, a dog ran in front of her and she fell, bracing herself with her left arm to protect her head. She broke her elbow in three places and had a hairline fracture of her humerus. She did intensive physical therapy for a year and was able to get back to playing, but when she came to see me, five years later, she was still experiencing pain in her arm and increasing stiffness. She was also feeling back stiffness and had a bunion on her left foot.

From my point of view, watching her walk, the whole left side had a diminished quality of movement.

I invited her to lie on the table on her back while suggesting she experiment with keeping a big frame of perception. I coached her to feel her head resting on the pillow, because when she was sitting and using her arms, I noticed how her head position and her way of holding her axis, or "center line," restricted the arm movement. As her head rested back on the pillow, she mentioned being reminded of how she loved to float in the ocean—the feeling of support.

I put my hand under hers and asked her to feel through her hand to mine underneath it as I invited her to follow my hand sliding towards the foot end of the table. Then I asked her to feel the table with the inside of her elbow and to let her elbow come out towards me.

Yes, these movements helped me investigate the range of motion of the shoulder, but there is more to it. I didn't think to myself, "I'm evaluating a shoulder joint's mobility." In my touch, I touch Rhea, as if I am touching her whole body at once. I meet a whole system, a whole person. This benefits me too: the quality of touch helps my own hand/arm/shoulder find the most stability. I keep my attention peripheral, listening. I remember how Hubert called the arm a "transitional organ"—a go-between from outside to inside and back.

> This way, the good coordination can come "exogenously" [from the out-side]. It's not a biomechanical question in the end; it's a relational question. Why with the arm? Because the arm is a transitional organ. It is built in the transitivity; it doesn't exist by itself.

Trying to explain what Hubert and I mean by calling the arm a transitional organ would not have worked for this session, but I suggested to Rhea that the hand is organized by the world and the arm connects us to each other.

With my hand still under hers, I asked her to start the movement with her arm extended, suggesting that she sense the connection with me and then begin a small twist of her torso, rotating away from me. I remember that she said she was imagining scar tissue growing in the space between her shoulder and her chest, and this restricted her movement. She asked me if the tissue needed to stretch—the mechanical view of the body. I encouraged the contact between our two hands, and then all of a sudden there were tears in her eyes—not because the movement hurt, but because something emotional welled up. Hubert credits François Delsarte (1811–1871) with calling the shoulder "the thermometer of emotion" (Stebbins, 1885). This was not a memory "stored" in the body. It was about reclaiming a possibility, *the missing gesture*—in this case, the sense of contact.

Rhea's tears, she said, had to do with feeling so alone during the time of her injury, as a single parent of two children who were quite young at that time. She tried to stifle the tears, although I reassured her, adding (for the cortex's reasoning ears) that tears release stress hormones. The emotion was almost a reflection of the missing gesture: reaching out in longing, receiving contact—what was not done, not expressed at the time.

It is very common for a small moment of release to arise when a pat-tern is changing. Hubert sometimes would call this welling up the "petit emotion." It is a moment that allows integration and movement, not at all the old model of catharsis. Rhea was surprised at her response, and very relieved, she said. Somehow her physical complaint made more sense when she was able to connect it to a movement in the present and her emotional experience of the past. The whole process opened up new pos-sibilities for her.

To end the session, I asked Rhea to come to standing, finding ease through the feet. When I tried the approach of giving some support to her head, she stiffened up. So instead, taking my cue from her responses, I suggested coming back to the feeling of the ocean around her, even in standing—the image of support that she had offered me at the beginning of the session.

I met with Rhea only that one time when she passed through Boston. Her session is a good example of the power of understanding the missing gesture. By starting from her physical injury and inviting a simple movement—opening—along with contact, she was able to reclaim the gesture of reaching, to feel the yearning from the time five years before when the problems began. The missing gesture was crucial for bringing movement to the stiffened area, but it had not been recognized as a necessary part of rehabilitation until our session.

EXPRESSIVE GESTURE

Imagine a picture of someone extending their arms in supplication, or a little child reaching up to a loved one, or someone pointing to show someone else, "Look!" All these gestures are an expression; they communicate a feeling, an interest, a shared perception, a relationship. This is part of what Hubert meant when he called the arm a "transitional organ."

The movement patterns of our arms are also established as we contact and use objects, from an infant's toys to a child's pencil and sports equipment. Over time, many varied experiences accumulate of handling, moving, and engaging with the objects of daily life. From the outside in, the ball shapes the baby's hand, and from the inside out, eventually the hand will be shaped in anticipation of catching the ball. That is another meaning of the arm as a "transitional organ."

The movement of our arms in gestures of expression is intimately connected with the functioning of shoulder, elbow, wrist joints, and hands. The way I touch or don't, the gestures that I allow or don't, directly impact the stability of the shoulder.

Yet if any of us experiences tension or pain or lack of flexibility in our arms and shoulders, it is immediately the mechanical aspect—muscles, joints, et cetera—that comes to mind. Strengthening, stretching, and surgical procedures are the go-to solutions to manage these problems.

We could think about our pain at least in part as a problem of expressive gesture just as much as mechanical overuse.

The expressive quality of arms is also a matter of personal significance to me. In 1981, I attended a pre-training for aspiring Rolfers called Perceptual Body in New York City. In the first meeting, we were videotaped walking towards the camera, introducing ourselves, turning, and walking away. At 21 years old, this was the first time I had seen myself on camera this way—in 1981, we were not used to seeing ourselves all the time! I was shocked at the sight of my arms, hanging limply by my sides. Was it the result of many years of training not to touch the antiques in my childhood home for fear of breaking something? Being told not to hang on people? A way of hiding? There may be many elements behind the shape I saw.

Hubert was the first teacher I met who stressed the key place of arms in our posture. Most approaches assume that the body is built from the ground up, like any other structure. "Grounding" and "rooting" are powerful images that represent important functions. But an often-disregarded dimension of finding the ground has to do with what lets go from above. The pattern of holding in the shoulders and arms has to begin to let go for us to be able to find grounding, just as much as the other way around. Often the shoulder pattern has to free up first, or it prevents anything else from changing.

The significance of the movements of our hands and arms goes deep: babies have a grasp reflex, an inheritance from when holding mom's fur was key to survival. They begin to reach for things before they can even sit on their own. Long before infants manage to sit up or walk independently, patterns of reaching for loved ones and objects, patterns of literally pushing, and metaphorically pushing away, are established. These patterns will be there when the child stands up. For all of us, the expressiveness of the arms, or lack thereof, is inevitably going to be connected to posture, and to others. *Transitive arms* are formed in relationship to an Other, formed in a personal and cultural context.

Hubert was fond of pointing out that in the shoulder joint, the socket for the humerus is very shallow compared to the hip joint. Rather than being primarily stabilized by thick ligaments the way the femur is in the hip socket, the shoulder's integrity is maintained in great part by the muscles called the "rotator cuff." Compared to ligaments, muscles come under the sway of our arousal system to a greater extent (Ribot-Ciscar *et al.*, 2000). This means that the arms and shoulders operate like a thermometer: responding to and reflecting our moment-to-moment emotional state, as well as the longer-term patterns we call "attitude." They don't release once and for all. Instead, we can use the arms' expressive quality as a doorway for practice.

EMBODIMENT: TRANSITIVITY

From the first workshops with Hubert, he emphasized the importance of our hands and arms in expression and in relating us to our surroundings. He had us work with a stick again, about the size of a closet dowel. This time, lying on our backs, the stick in our hands, he said to the class: "First, let yourself notice where you and the stick are touching. Notice the place of contact—it is a two-way process: you are touching the stick and being touched by the stick at the same time."

With this quality of contact, the stick floated up, taking one joint of the upper limb at a time—only the fingers, then the palms, then the wrists (carpal bones), then radius, then ulna, then humerus, and then scapula—each joint articulating between ground and sky. As described in the Introduction, touching the stick and letting in the touch of the stick changed so much in my physical experience. Instead of grasping, there was contact, a meeting that continued to be a process of discovery, never resolving into the habitual, what is known and expected.

In the modified Sun Salutation with our hands on a chair, which he called "Flight of the Eagle," Hubert engaged us in practices that involved working with mechanical and expressive qualities simultaneously. We explored how we met the surfaces we contacted, how we were able or not to expand into the surrounding space. He never asked us to "raise our arms," but instead it was always with an imaginative framing: as if we had our best friends on either side and we were reaching for them, or projecting out into the space far away, or greeting the sun.

Hubert described the arm as the place where the missing gesture—"the gestures that I do not allow myself"—is perhaps most likely to show up, because "it is linked with expression/impression." He went on: "It is a gate to go from inside to outside" (H. Godard, personal communication, November 24, 2009). This gives context to Hubert's cryptic saying that the arms are transitive. Go-betweens. They are often telling a story. It could be important to be in conversation with clients, while we work together, to give people space to let me know their associations or what is coming up. But even without that, it's important to bear the arms' complexity in mind.

In this somatic approach, there is simultaneously a physical impact and a change on another level. The muscles do get stronger; coordination and balance do improve. But these changes are a consequence or at least go together with a change in the other layers of perception, body image, expression, and symbolic gesture.

In the model where muscles are given the primary importance, a person might be told to strengthen the serratus anterior muscle, the primary stabilizer of the shoulder blade. Sometimes a little bodybuilding of specific muscles is useful: the movements involved in waking up serratus anterior bring about a kinesthetic change. This reintroduces the option of recruiting those particular fibers. Like musicians in an orchestra at the ready, they are available to play the kinetic melody. But reclaiming the potential of action is far more than serratus anterior, or triceps, or any muscle. What is reclaimed is a sense of actions possible in an environment.

When I was working with Rhea, it was the quality of my contact, what Hubert calls "haptic capacity," that helped stabilize my own shoulder blade. If I had been touching Rhea with distaste, or in a more objectifying way, instead of the quality of my hand's contact helping to recruit my own serratus anterior fibers, I would be more likely to trigger my large forearm muscles in a grasp, with no give and take in the hand itself. Serratus would miss its chance; instead, my pectoralis minor would probably have worked first, pulling my shoulder blade out of its optimum mechanical position for stability.

I am going into these details to show that our attitudes cannot be separated from our mechanics. Mechanics express an attitude; they manifest it. Not just a personal one, but one that is imbued with cultural overlay. They are at once our most personal expression and a reflection of our society.

"THROWING LIKE A GIRL"

There is a long history of the significance of gesture, Hubert explained at a workshop in Montreux, Switzerland, in 2009. The classic example is in the movement of throwing: a hundred years ago, it was noticed that many women could not throw. Instead, they in a sense *pushed* the ball, with no rotation of the trunk or leaning back. One of the most well-known studies of this phenomenon is Iris Marion Young's 1980 essay "Throwing like a girl," which addressed the issue of the embodied experience of gender from a feminist point of view.

Hubert paraphrased de Beauvoir: "You are not born a woman, you become one." The fact that many women don't automatically find the gesture of throwing has nothing to do with physiology; it is a social mold that is imposed from the outside. Young argued that societal expectations and structures shaped the way women inhabit their bodies, often limiting their physical agency and confidence. She called for greater awareness of how societal frameworks shape not only behavior but also the fundamental ways individuals experience and express themselves in the world. It is remarkable that something as seemingly innocuous as throwing a ball—such a mundane movement—could from an early age reflect a girl's sense of self, of possibilities.

Hubert gave us the example of male and female fashion models at the time to make the point. He described how male models walked on the runway like Marlon Brando, "arms rotated internally, like a gorilla." The women, in contrast, frequently walked as if their arms were pinned between the shoulder blades, with the teres major muscles held in external rotation (teres major runs between the shoulder blade and the humerus). Hubert pointed out that this pre-movement prevents the freedom to move into punching or throwing. This is an example of the missing gesture. To change the pre-movement in this case, he said, "When you put the shoulder girdle back on its axis, you open the possibility of new gestures and new capacities of expression."

TAI CHI ARMS

I can attest to this. Early in my work with Hubert, a colleague offered a portrayal of my arms as *geworfen*—flung into the world, limp and passive, as I described before. These days, Hubert's ideas come back to me regularly in my practice of tai chi. What actions are permitted, and which are forbidden or avoided? How does that connect to the freedom of hands, arms, and shoulders in movement? To our posture and balance? All these themes are present.

My teacher, Don Miller,[1] does not teach a form of 24 or any number. His approach is to delve into each move, so the students can discover the endless relationships each move can express. I think of the practices as variations on a theme. Take the movements of "Grasp Sparrow's Tail," for example, translated as ward off, roll back, press, and push. Each one is an expression of a particular quality. Ward off is a way of expanding into self-protection instead of tensing. Roll back is release without collapse. Press can be more like condensation, becoming more dense, rather than fear, tension, or aggression. Push can bring in all those qualities for strength without effortful contraction. It is a practice of transformation. To find each of the qualities reflected in Grasp Sparrow's Tail is a way to practice a series of pre-movements, in which sensations and imagination precede the visible gesture. How do we expand in all directions at once for ward off? How does letting go in roll back become a form of strength? Of course, being able to maintain a connection with heaven and earth, what Don calls "rooting" and "rising," has to be included in each gesture. This foundational pre-movement is the capacity to orient to ground and sky while exploring new gestures. Don's approach to tai chi is a beautiful expression of Hubert's understanding of movement.

Don likes to bring in quite a variety of qualities: we can use free flow and fling our arms in the movements of Grasp Sparrow's Tail, and then do the moves with bound flow, carefully carving each moment, agonists and antagonists engaged.[2] We can emphasize the dragon, the spiraling quality of the hands, limbs, spine, folding and twisting inwards and outwards. And sometimes we do all the gestures with fists—tai chi fists—which spiral in and don't engage a big biceps contraction.

I find that the practice of varying the arms' quality leads to better orientation, freeing the central axis, the spine becoming tai chi's strand of pearls, hanging from the sky. It is the variation that leads to a strong central line. With so many transformations, the arms have to let go of any postural activity. Then the sense of two directions, extending beyond the head, beyond the floor, provides a new way to manage instability. And in addition, I am invited into the domain of missing gestures.

In my normal life, I never punch. I rarely have a reason to make a fist. At first, doing so in tai chi class really felt forbidden. Now, at the end of the sessions, I feel like a heavyweight boxer or the male fashion models with the strong arms Hubert had described. The thought is: "Very unladylike." Luckily, I have practice with allowing those thoughts and the associated feelings. The autonomic nervous system gets activated and engenders a vagal response—sweating, heat rising, sometimes trembling. The energy spent in avoiding certain gestures begins to move. A small charge arises as the gestures unconsciously forbidden are finally allowed. In Hubert's words:

These muscles are also the defense of territory. It's not nothing: I can push you away, and I can say no; once you have found the way to organize the core, you have a lot of strength. When you have that force, even a fragile person can push. It's a new experience.

It's not nothing! As Hubert described it, reclaiming gestures is reclaiming possible actions along with their implications. The new possibilities have to be metabolized. What if I enjoy punching? What arises when I feel dangerous?

In tai chi, after each practice, there is a chance to digest the arousal in *wu chi*, empty standing. Just standing. Feeling the ground and the surrounding space all the way to the sky. The reactivity has a chance to dissolve. Over time the movements are more familiar, and even fun. It gives different meaning to "range of motion"—more like "range of expression." It's not that I need to literally punch: what has been reclaimed is the *possibility* of the missing gesture.

INSTRUMENTAL AND EXPRESSIVE GESTURE

Hubert mentioned at the class in Chandolin, Switzerland, in 2008 that there is a difference between what he called *instrumental movements*—such as lifting a weight in an exercise or grasping a pen—and *expressive gestures*—when we open our arms for a hug or talk with our hands. Philosopher Sean Gallagher notes that expressive gesture is linked to language and proposes: "that gesture is not a form of instrumental action but a form of expressive action; not a reproduction of an original instrumental behavior but a different kind of action altogether" (Gallagher, 2005, p.117). He suggests that gesture "is part of and is controlled by a linguistic/communicative system rather than a motor system" (Gallagher, 2005, p.118).

Gallagher reports the surprising example of children who are blind from birth, who therefore have never seen anything at all, but still gesture with their hands when they talk, even when they are speaking with someone who is also blind. Without having ever seen anyone else, their gestures still resemble those of a sighted person. The blind children's expressive gestures support Gallagher's point that the movements that come from expression may even be generated in a different part of the brain than the instrumental ones. He quotes French philosopher Maurice Merleau-Ponty (1908–1961): "language *accomplishes* thought" (Gallagher,

2005, p.121). Gesture communicates to others, but it also may serve our own understanding, our own cognition, as we shape our thoughts.

Hubert sums all this up when he says, "You need your arm to think." Expressive gestures have something to do with language and they have something to do with mind. It is as if the gestures are a part of language, and language is movement. Both are expressive: they are inherently related, and inherently different from pragmatic, deliberate, controlled gestures.

I was reminded of the beautiful movement of the little three-year-old children in a Duncan Dance performance I attended years ago. Rather than instruct them about how to move, the teacher came on stage and reached into the pouch attached to her belt. Pulling out a handful of white feathers, she threw them up in the air, and the children with one breath said, "Ahhh," reaching up in unison to catch the feathers as they floated down—movement as expression and response. When we see our shoulder problems only in terms of mechanics, we miss this whole important dimension—the human experience—arms moving, expressing, responding, in relationship to the world we encounter.

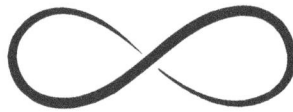

We have come a long way from the image of body displayed in the Body Worlds exhibits. Hubert's model of integration links our physical structure with our movement patterns—coordination—and follows Gibson in considering perception as a skill. The dimension of meaning, metaphor, the symbolic—what calls us and what we avoid—cannot be divorced from the need to manage in a terrestrial environment, to orient in the gravitational field. Body reading includes all these dimensions. Skill building begins with gravity, context, and through our perception of this most basic of polarities—two directions, two ways of sensing gravity, up and down, heaven and earth.

To develop a reliable body, all these aspects will need to be included: we can't separate our symptoms from our psyche, our physical experience from our experience of meaning, and all of it is in an encounter with our surroundings which always include our perception of weight and space.

What else is involved in perceiving? That is the topic of Part III.

PART III

PERCEIVING

CHAPTER TEN

A Sense for Movement

Now that we can imagine perception as a skill, how do we go about exercising it? Part III explores the language and landscape of perception, examining familiar and unfamiliar terms, such as body awareness, body schema, and proprioception, among others. Considering the role of vision and separating the strands of sensation and perception are also important. As the array of terms is disentangled, it allows us to refine our language and invites us to become more perceptive.

SY—SEEKING BODY AWARENESS

Sy, a man in his mid-20s, walks into my office. From the shape of the muscles defining his shoulders under his T-shirt, I can see that he's athletic. He's here for his first session of Rolfing and Movement Integration. I invite him to sit in the chair by my desk. "What's bringing you in here today?" I ask.

He tells me he was a three-season athlete throughout high school and college—football, basketball, and track and field. Now he just lifts weights, what he calls *training*.

"My body is a mess!" he tells me and begins to list his injuries: he took a bad fall years ago when his legs were cut out from under him while playing basketball, and his back still hurts. He attributes the chronic pain in his shoulder to throwing javelin in competitions. He has sprained his ankles, rolling them many times. He's not playing anything anymore. He imagined weightlifting would help him heal, but the old injuries still plague him. "How can I get this body back to feeling good?" he asks. "I'm ready to try something different!"

As he talks, I listen and notice the impression he makes on me. He looks strong and buff. The outer shape of his body is defined, like shoulder pads or armor. He presents the picture of an athletic bodybuilder. The bulked-up muscles are a sign of strength, but what Sy tells me is a story of vulnerability. It's as if his outward strength masks the weakness he is experiencing from his injuries. He's a big tough guy doing everything he can to strengthen his muscles, but he still has a sore shoulder and an aching back, and he's afraid he'll roll his ankles again.

The paradox of looking strong while feeling injured is the basis for an important distinction: the layer of muscles we can see may give someone the picture of muscular definition, but it is not the whole story when it comes to real strength. It is the task of deeper muscles and connective tissues—invisible to the eye—to support the joints and maintain posture. Dr. Rolf wrote about this distinction using the terms "core" and "sleeve" (Feitis, 1978, p.211). In Sy, we see an imbalance in which the outer, mostly bigger muscles (the sleeve) are built up to the detriment of the postural and support system (the core). This is common when there has been an emphasis on weightlifting. The imbalance is what I want to work with.

The difference in muscular activity is also a difference in Sy's perceptual choice. He sits forward in the chair, his feet crossed under the seat, barely touching the floor. I ask, "What is supporting you right now? What's stopping you from falling over?" In that posture, it takes a lot of extra effort to hold up his own body weight. What I'm looking for, what I'm not seeing, is the sense that he could take in the actual support the chair could give him, to have a chance to rest—to make a different perceptual choice.

Sense of support can be hard to describe, but it is easy to demonstrate. How much weight can you lift? That's the usual test, but I do a different one: "Why don't you stand up," I invite him. "How do you feel you should stand? What is good form for you?"

He tries to catch a glimpse in the mirror. He straightens up and squares his shoulders, pulling them back and lifting his chest, and tilts his chin down. This is what we tend to think good posture looks like, seen from the outside. Not quite military posture, but it looks like a lot of work!

He's taller than I am, and heavier, and I'm sure he can deadlift a lot more weight, but I put one hand behind him and with the other hand, I give a little push in the center of his chest. He staggers backwards, thrown off balance. He is "taken aback," surprised. (I'm used to this, which is why I kept my other hand behind him.)

This is a useful experiment to help someone understand what "aligned in gravity" means. A sense of good support doesn't come from looking

good in the mirror, and it doesn't come from tension and effort. Good support is a feeling of solidity, often discovered by letting go of unnecessary
tension, as we have explored in the embodiments in previous chapters
(Chapter Three: *What and Where in practice*; Chapter Five: *What prevents
me?*).

Sy does what many people do: he looks to the mirror to find his good
form. It's a common misconception that good posture is what you look
like. He comes by this understanding honestly: today we see so many
images of ourselves! It's natural to refer to these images when we look for
ourselves—to see how we stand, what position we're in, how we feel. We
may look for these images in the mirror or our imagination, remembering
what worked before.

In the process of putting himself in the right place visually, Sy contracts
many muscles, creating tensions that lift up his body weight, making him
top-heavy and actually weakening him. His posture might look right to
him in the mirror, but the holding and tensions shift him off his center
of gravity. He may feel straight, but he's off balance, easy to push over.

Why doesn't he feel off balance without my help? Why doesn't he
instinctively choose the most mechanically efficient strategy for his body?
The problem is not unique to him. Although most of us have no problem
getting around or standing up, for example, we don't automatically know
how our bodies are relating to gravity or to our surroundings. We don't
feel this aspect of what we do or how we do it. We mostly feel the consequences, like stiffness or pain, of choices we don't realize we are making.
Then we may try to impose a correction effortfully, as Sy did when he
tightened his shoulders to stand up "straight."

When I ask him to let his weight rest into the ground, I see that his
feet are not giving him good support. When the weight reaches his feet,
instead of landing on an arch that can spring, it shifts inward. He reminds
me: "I can't tell you the number of times that I have rolled those ankles!" I
see why he would unconsciously hold himself up; letting go into his feet
is almost an experience of collapse.

Who is making this decision? Sy's system perceived an instability and
chose a strategy—to hold himself up by the shoulders—at least in part
because the alternative—letting his weight down—doesn't give him a feeling of support. He holds himself up by his shoulders over ankles that roll
way too easily and feet that fall instead of springing. As practitioners, it is
important to recognize the individual differences in strategy for maintaining equilibrium before we offer a solution. For instance, asking Sy to get

more grounded wouldn't help him let go of the tension in his shoulders. In his case, his body/mind is taking a logical approach to managing ankle instability, by holding himself up from above. Still, those shoulders he has built up with weight training are sustaining him at a price. His shoulder injury can't heal while he overuses his shoulder muscles to keep himself upright.

Is there hope that he can feel better? Yes, there is. In addition to strengthening, soft tissue work can help his feet and ankles, and in the meantime, I can help him shift his perceptions. Instead of putting the focus on his feet meeting the ground, I hold the back of his head, the nape of the neck where the base of the cranium meets the first cervical vertebra, and I ask him to walk. I invite him to let go, to hang from there, because as we saw with Fred Astaire's style, the feeling of support can also come from above.

Sy's predicament reflects a common problem: how to work with our body to feel less pain, instead of struggling against it. What do we do when working hard to hold ourselves upright doesn't help and when looking in the mirror to try to find the right posture doesn't work either? We aren't usually taught that our comfort and ease depend on a nuanced relationship with gravity, or that we can use perceptual cues to change preconscious choices, as Sy could use the message from my touch on the back of his neck to relax his whole body. Anyone who finds their way into my office has an effective strategy for staying up in gravity, but that doesn't mean it is a sustainable one. Usually, what brings people to the office are the unintended consequences of unconscious strategies that are based in perceptual choices. But new options are available! There is enormous potential for each one of us in taking this different viewpoint. As I learned in Hubert's classes, we can start again with every movement, in every moment.

TERMS OF EMBODIMENT

People often ascribe their symptoms to bad posture or a lack of body awareness. But what is body awareness? And how do we improve it? It is not enough to tell someone to stand up straight. That doesn't work; it leads to the holding we so often see. As we saw in Sy's example, some part of him that was not entirely conscious made decisions about his posture.

Can we influence these decisions? What do we need to understand to help ourselves or others?

TRY THIS   ✓

Pause for just a moment. What are you experiencing right now as you come into the present? The sense of the chair giving you support? The floor under your feet? The surrounding space, with its light and its sounds? Do you notice the movement of the breath? And the next breath...

When people come to my office and I ask them what they are noticing, often they respond, "I don't know," or they tell me what hurts: "I can't turn my head." "My knee hurts when I walk down the stairs." Or they repeat what someone else said: "My chiropractor says I have one leg longer than the other." "My wife tells me I slouch." "I see myself in the mirror and one shoulder is higher than the other." We are not accustomed to describing the experience of sensing. Aside from pain that really gets our attention, we often seem entirely oblivious of the perceptual information upon which our movements and much more depend. Are we oblivious or do we lack the language to express what we perceive in this moment? Research shows that a key aspect of emotional intelligence is being able to describe our feelings with more complexity (Kashdan *et al.*, 2015). That necessitates having words in our vocabulary that allow us to perceive and distinguish what we are feeling. I have found the same to be true for somatic intelligence: we need to expand and develop the terms we use in order to capture the complex dimensions behind the popular idea of body awareness. How do we understand embodiment? Where will we find words?

BODY IMAGE/BODY SCHEMA

Since the 19th century, physiologists (and later psychologists and neuroscientists) have investigated problems with body perception, seeking an understanding of their patients who show changes in bodily experience related to disease, limb loss, or neurological incidents such as strokes. In 1911, two British neurologists, Sir Henry Head and Gordon Holmes, studied people with brain damage that impacted their body sense, cases called spatial neglect. These patients might shave only one side of their face, or dress only one side of their body. (We consider the spatial aspect of neglect in depth in Chapter Fifteen: Action Space.) In their paper, Head and Holmes distinguished two sides of the problem: one they called "body image" and the other "body or postural schema." They defined body image as "an internal representation in the conscious experience of visual, tactile and motor information of corporal origin," (cited in Paillard, 1999, p.197) and body schema as "a combined standard against which all subsequent changes of posture are measured...before they enter consciousness" (Head & Holmes, 1911, p.187). Head and Holmes postulated the body schema as an internal model of body posture, a neural representation that would serve as a stand-in for the body-in-the-world and would allow the brain to plan and predict movement. Head and Holmes' definitions base the distinction between the two concepts on accessibility to consciousness (body image) in contrast to pre-, sub-, or unconscious processes (body schema).

Head and Holmes' terms—body schema and body image—are still widely used, and their work has been cited thousands of times (Sattin *et al.*, 2023). A hundred years of research has led to clarification, but also confusion. Today we know that body schema does not arise from just one brain area. It includes many processes—multiple brain regions, receptors, perceptual information, the state of the body, the sense of location, et cetera—that allow us to keep track of where we are as we move. When we take a closer look, our body sense is neither simple nor straightforward, and the distinction between conscious processes and unconscious ones is less clear.

In 1995, Shaun Gallagher (the philosopher mentioned in Chapter Nine) and Jonathan Cole, a medical doctor, attempted to disentangle Head and Holmes's concepts in their paper, "Body Image and Body Schema in a Deafferented Subject" (Gallagher & Cole, 2001). *Afferent* refers to the signals that come from the periphery to the brain, often termed "sensory." The deafferented patient, Ian Waterman, had lost these signals. In other words, Ian's body schema had lost access to primary information needed to guide movement. Surprisingly, over time Ian found a way to control his movement again, primarily by using deliberate effort to guide his visual image of his body. Gallagher and Cole's paper detailed how body image and schema worked together in Ian's case, to help us understand more of the complexity of body awareness.

When Hubert asked us to read this paper, I remember wondering what was important about Ian Waterman's experience and the terminology used to describe it. Over time, I understood that the terms reflect a helpful and still evolving conceptual framework for understanding—and hence working with—movement. They highlight the complex reality behind our capacity to "just do it," as Nike's slogan goes (Nike, 1988). Because how do we "just do it"? How do we plan action? How do we know where we are? I found that expanding my frame of reference to include many aspects of the movement system helped me influence my own movement patterns more effectively. But to understand all this for myself, I first had to delve into the details of Ian Waterman's experience.

IAN'S STORY[1]

When Ian Waterman woke up in the hospital, he couldn't feel his body. The 19-year-old had cut his finger while working as an apprentice in a butcher shop and came down with a flu-like virus shortly after, but no one expected this: he couldn't feel his body or the bed where he lay. His speech was slurred. The admitting doctor's first impression was that Ian was drunk, but by the morning it was clear that something was seriously wrong. For his predicament to be ascribed to a night on the town was the first of many painful misunderstandings Ian experienced as he struggled to make sense of his new condition.

For the first few weeks, Ian was completely helpless. He still could not feel his body. His speech became clearer, but his tongue remained numb. It wasn't that moving was impossible: his limbs could move, but he had no control over them. Early on after his illness, if he turned to speak to someone on his right side, his left arm might float up or knock something off the nightstand. Moving not only felt useless but also dangerous.

Ian had lost the sense of where his body was. What was going on? An inability to control movement could be caused by brain damage, which would prevent the brain from sending a message to the muscles, or if the spinal cord itself has been damaged, the neurological message could be interrupted. Yet Ian wasn't paralyzed, but rather lacked sensation. His brain was no longer getting feedback through his nervous system about where his body was, so he couldn't control his movements. Rather than his brain failing to send messages to his limbs, the interruption was occurring in the other direction: the peripheral nerves that transmit sensory information to the brain had been permanently damaged.[2]

Ian's experience brings home how much we take for granted about movement. Textbooks tend to use a simple anatomical motor/sensory distinction: motor commands go out from the brain, sensory messages come in from the periphery. Ian's experience shows that, functionally, motor and sensory cannot be neatly separated. Ian's motor system was intact, but without sensory input, he couldn't control his movement. In the terms used by Head and Holmes, Ian's body schema—his brain's representation of his body—was no longer receiving updates from the receptors embedded in muscle and joints, his proprioceptors. Ian's doctors could identify what had happened to his nervous system, but they had no idea what it would mean for his recovery.

Most of us have intact nervous systems, but as we saw with Sy, we too "lose our bodies." We imagine that we are controlling our movements, but the body seems to have a mind of its own (Blakeslee & Blakeslee, 2007). Can we learn something about our own embodiment from Ian's experience?

LOSING YOUR BODY, LOSING YOUR BALANCE

After a few weeks and little improvement, Ian was moved from the hospital to a rehabilitation center nearby. As Ian recounts it:

> I vividly remember the journey from Jersey to the Neurological Centre. Until then I had been safely cocooned in hospital, cosseted and fussed over. The journey brought home to me the extent of my problem. I can remember sitting, propped up in the corner of the ambulance. At the first bend I found myself falling over and was just saved by the ambulance man from injuring myself. I had no balance. I didn't move in time and sympathy with the vehicle. I couldn't respond and save myself from falling. I suddenly realized I had no effective control over my body. I became very confused and frightened. (Cole, 1995, p.18)

Who would think that riding in a car requires enormous feedback and communication between our sense receptors to our brains and back to maintain our balance? Balancing seems automatic, but we were not born with this ability. The engineers' attempts to build mobile robots, described in Chapter Two, shows that we don't realize all that is involved in keeping our balance—our orientation—as we go about our day. Ian describes a rare experience: when all these automatic, though partially learned, coordinated actions don't function. He didn't lose the motor programs, but rather the communication from his body's sensors to his brain. His body schema was not getting the information it needed to coordinate weight shift and ongoing movement. We don't usually think about how the information we get from the world provides essential support for all our movements. We tend to think of these as independent functions, when under normal circumstances they depend on each other—perception and action always intertwining.

KINESTHESIA: THE SIXTH SENSE

Like the falling down robots described previously, Ian's case reveals a critical aspect of understanding our own embodiment. The damage to Ian's nerves robbed him of the ability to feel touch below his neck, and it also took away something less obvious: what Cole describes as the sixth sense, kinesthesia—the subconscious awareness of the body and joints.

Distinguishing proprioception and kinesthesia

The term *kinesthesis* was coined in 1887 by H. C. Bastian, an English medical researcher, to designate "the sense of movement"—"the body of sensations which result from or are directly occasioned to movement" (Bastian, 1887, p.5). Two decades later, Charles Sherrington (1857–1952), Nobel Prize–winning physiologist, adopted the term *proprioception* to describe the perception of joint and body movement, as well as position of the body, or body segments, in space (Sherrington, 1906). Sherrington was one of the first to investigate the influence of sensory connections on the control of movement and posture, and he included both in his use of proprioception. The terms kinesthesia and proprioception are often used interchangeably in research contexts. However, as we continue, we may find it useful to distinguish between them.

"Posture accompanies movement like its shadow," Sherrington wrote in 1932 (Creed *et al.*, 1938, quoted in Stuart, 2005, pp.624–625). Contemporary neuroscience research affirms the existence of two distinct senses: proprioception is the sense of the body's position detected by joint receptors, whereas kinesthesia refers specifically to the ability to sense the extent and direction of movement through muscle spindles and skin stretch receptors (Proske & Gandevia, 2009). Ian lost both kinds of receptors—for position sense and for movement. For now, we will use both terms to designate Ian's perceptual loss. This constant stream of information from muscles, joints, and skin that keep us aware of our movements and posture abruptly disappeared after Ian's illness. For practical purposes, in our daily movement, can we truly distinguish between proprioception and kinesthesia? Are we ever truly still? Staying upright depends on a subconscious conversation between gravity's signals of weight shift, our receptors, and the representation our brain makes of this information. As Ian's recounting of riding in the ambulance shows, we need this information predictively for movement—before we move.

Kinesthesia, though often overlooked, is crucial to our ability to move (Cole, 1995, p.32). The flow of information you and I receive about where we are, which is constantly updated as our breath moves in and out, as our body shifts in its chair, as the winds around us change—this is what Ian was cut off from. Although we rarely think to exercise our kinesthetic sense per se,[3] a body in motion normally depends on it. It mostly happens without our conscious attention. As the mobile—or falling—robots illustrate, our kinesthetic sense is much less straightforward than it may appear. As Jaxon, the valve-turning robot showed us, perceiving the valve, knowing you have it in your grasp, and not falling over when you turn it is a complex problem. What light can neuroscience research shed?

In the past, doctors such as Head and Holmes, confronted with body sense troubles in patients with brain damage, came up with the concept of body schema or postural schema to describe what the patients were experiencing trouble *with.* But Ian's brain was not damaged. In his case, his doctors could identify the specific nerves that were destroyed by the virus, but they had no idea what Ian was experiencing and didn't know how to help him. If he had lost the neural pathways controlling his movements, they might have prescribed motion exercises to foster the growth of new pathways, but Ian had not had a stroke; he wasn't paralyzed, and this approach would not work for him. Ian struggled to put into words what was wrong, what was missing, what he had to do in order to find a way to move again. He was on his own.

Even though it is so important, kinesthesia is a subconscious process for us. We are mostly unaware of its contribution to movement. For example, Sy didn't arrive at my office saying something was wrong with his kinesthetic sense or that his body schema needed help. He assumed his symptoms reflected weakness and mechanical failure. Ian's story, however, helps us begin to articulate how kinesthesia goes on in the background and how we might work with this sense ourselves.

In our conscious relationship to our remarkable ability to move, we are very much like children who, every day, bring their dirty dishes into the kitchen and put them in the sink. The children, busy with their toys or their next entertainment, don't have to be concerned about how the dishes get cleaned—someone else takes care of this. Laundry, grocery shopping, and other mundane tasks of daily life go on, but the children are more or less oblivious. That is how we relate to our ability to move. We're mostly oblivious.

Right now, as you read these words, you are sitting or standing (hence, not falling over) or lying down, managing to hold the book or device you are using without dropping it. All of this depends on your capacity for kinesthesia. To hold the book, your brain has to perceive it. That process happens partly through receptors in your skin, joints, and muscles, which transmit information that is processed in the brain. At the same time, you must also not fall over, and that's another job your brain and perceptual systems are taking care of at this very moment. Your system has its own experience of you as a body. This experience is shaping you, but you probably don't realize it. Just like a competent parent who helps our lives run smoothly, every moment a wealth of neurological signals is combined into a representation we are here calling "body schema." This is not an abstraction; it is happening right now.

TRY THIS

Take a moment to notice your kinesthetic sense right now. There is a breath. You are inhaling or exhaling, filling or emptying. You are breathing, and you aren't falling over. You are able to maintain your uprightness in relation to the field of gravity that surrounds you while being moved by the breath. Everything else you do depends on this!

Information about your state of being, where you are, what is supporting you, the various forces that are acting on you—all causing sensations in receptor sites at various places in the body—combine to create the system's body schema. From this complex stream of signals, decisions about balance and movement are selected. As long as it works for us, we can be oblivious. It takes the courage of someone like Ian sharing the story of his loss and its consequences to help us understand this aspect of embodiment: what our body schema does for us.

REHABILITATION AND ADAPTATION

It is hard to imagine what it felt like to be Ian after his illness. It took him four months and a lot of careful planning, immense effort, and practice to be able to even sit up in bed. It would be a year before he could come to his feet and stand. When he showed his neurologist, Dr. Graveson, that he had mastered standing on crutches for 40 minutes, the pessimistic doctor didn't even react. The neurological tests showed no improvement in nerve function, blinding the doctor to what standing up meant to Ian: a significant recovery of function and agency.

In one sense, Dr. Graveson was right: Ian never regained function of the receptors most of us take for granted. But the doctor misjudged Ian's will, and the remarkable adaptability of our movement system. Ian was determined to figure out a way to move independently.

Ian never lost control of his head movements. His vestibular system was intact, giving him the ability to know which way was up. Ian's trouble was from the neck down. Jonathan Cole, Ian's doctor and biographer, speculates that, along with his determination, the preservation of his vestibular capacity and the very important navigational information it supplies were key to Ian's ability to reclaim function. Cole also attributes it to the fact that Ian's illness occurred when he was 19 years old: old enough to have established many motor programs and to have familiarity with the way movements feel, but young enough to have the strength and motivation to continue to strive for better function.

An example of neuroplasticity

The doctors knew that Ian had lost skin sensation and the sensations from joints and muscles that convey where the limbs are in space. In addition, the virus had knocked out all of Ian's muscle spindles below the neck: the tiny, specialized fiber bundles that are sensitive to stretch. Generally, the muscle spindles respond to the changes in length of the muscle, thereby communicating information to the nervous system about the position of arms and legs and how we are moving. The estimated 20,000–50,000 spindles are not evenly distributed: they are present in greater density in locations that are important for feedback such as the neck, since stabilizing the inner ear and the eyes is so vitally important. Ian's illness did not affect his head and neck, but it destroyed the nerves sending information from all the other receptors in joints and tendons and spindles throughout his body.

Fiber Type	Myelinated						Unmyelinated	
Conduction Velocity, m/s	120	90	60	30	6	2	2	0.5
Diameter, Microns	20	15	10	5	1	2	2	0.5

Sensory Receptor and [Perception]:

muscle spindles
tendon receptors
[joint position sense]
[proprioception]
[muscle stretch]

cutaneous receptors
[touch]
[proprioception]

subcutaneous pressure receptors
[deep pressure]

nociceptors
[sharp pain]

thermoreceptors
[cold]

thermoreceptors
[warmth]

nociceptors
[dull pain]

small muscle receptors
[tension]
[cramp]
[fatigue]
[effort]

Table 1: Schematic diagram of the types and functions
of the peripheral nerves (Cole, 1995)
*The nerves in bold are the ones that Ian lost. Proprioception—position sense
(joint receptors)—and kinesthesia—movement sense (muscle spindles and skin
stretch receptors); muscle spindle primary endings can contribute to both.*

Table 1 above shows the peripheral nerves that Ian lost in bold type. The table also shows smaller receptors that respond to deep pressure and sharp pain. Receptors called *free nerve endings* are sensitive to dull pain, warmth, and muscle fatigue. Lacking the fast-conducting fatty myelin sheath,[4] these nerves convey sensory information more slowly than the larger myelinated nerves that innervate muscle spindles and tendon receptors. These receptors were not impacted by the virus.

Over time, Ian began to find new ways to locate his body using these different channels of perceptual information. Since he couldn't see his body under the covers when he woke up in the morning, he didn't immediately know how his body was located. To find himself, he had to use subtler cues: a sense of cold, for example, might alert him to where his leg was, or if he heard a bump, that would signal to him that a limb had moved. No new sensation might mean that one leg had gotten stuck under the other. Deep touch and temperature could act as some compensation for the missing spindle information (Cole, 1995, p.84).

Usually, we would not need to take the time to locate ourselves through small temperature differences in our limbs. The signals from peripheral nerves to the brain are fast: if you touch a point in your wrist, 20 milliseconds later your cortex registers a response. Ian had lost this source of information, but he began to pick up the much slower signals from the small, myelinated fibers (A-delta). The response took 84 milliseconds: more than four times as long. Still, Ian was adapting to his new situation.

Ian is a rare case: in our daily lives, the movement system operates seamlessly, and we don't realize that we are using many channels of perception as we go about our daily lives. Through Ian's story, we are beginning to get to know the body schema and all it is responsible for as we move about the world. We will follow Ian's story into the next chapter to explore how he was able to use his visual perception, the conscious sense of body image, to find a way to move again.

TRY THIS
Perceptual channels
As we go about our day, we are tuning into different channels of sensory information essential for orientation, movement capacity, and our survival. Generally, we go around unaware of our choices and so our selection can become habitual, overusing some channels and underutilizing others. However, by guiding our awareness and paying attention differently, we can expand and refine our sensory channels. Follow the directions below to find out for yourself.
    Come to standing. If you feel comfortable, close your eyes.
    Gradually shift your weight towards the front half of your feet.

Pause to notice the sense of more pressure in your forefoot. This is registered by a variety of pressure-sensitive mechanoreceptors located in the soles of your feet.

Gradually increase your forward direction; what you feel in your calves is the effect of muscle spindles reacting to the imbalance. They are sensitive to stretch and set in motion the reflexes leading to muscle contractions that keep you from falling forward.

Notice your full body sense as you bring your weight back "home."

Guide your awareness to your skin, noticing the temperature of the air in your room—perhaps sunshine streams through your window or there is a cool breeze. These are your thermoreceptors registering temperature variations.

Raise your arms slowly upwards towards the sky and back down again. Explore moving one arm at a time and both arms at the same time; perhaps they move in different directions and shapes. Tune into the sense of your arms moving and your whole body adapting to this movement—the shifting that naturally happens in your knees, feet, and hips as you move your arms. This is kinesthesia at work.

Pause with one arm in a position in space. Notice the relationship of your hand to your elbow. Did you pause with your arm bent, straight, or in between? This is your sense of proprioception telling you about this position in space.

Gently open your eyes and notice where your arms are located—any surprises? Does your visual sense correspond with your felt sense with your eyes closed?

CHAPTER ELEVEN

Visual Kinesthesia

Ian Waterman has shown his generous spirit by spending hours with researchers. His personal struggle has been of great benefit to the rest of us in understanding embodiment. Having permanently lost the nerves that are usually used for proprioception and kinesthesia, Ian discovered that for more complex movement, his vision could substitute to some extent for the missing sensations. If he could see his limbs, he had some control over them—but only when they were in view. After a year in a rehabilitation facility, Ian went to live with his mother. In that apartment, they paid for electricity by the shilling, fed into a slot. One day, Ian was standing in the kitchen when the electricity cut out. The lights went out, and he fell down immediately. Vision was the only sense giving him feedback. Without it, he could not stay upright. Now, his mother says, they pay quarterly!

To this day, Ian needs to be able to see his body to know where he is. He needs light at all times, even when he is sleeping—if he woke in the dark, he would be lost without light. Because Ian's capacities are not based on neurological improvement, to this day he will still fall down if the lights go out. This man who can't feel his body can walk, but only with incredible effort and by using his vision. His visual system is active all the time when he is moving—as active as yours would be if you were juggling five balls at once. He is truly moving himself from the outside.

How do we *find* ourselves, those of us without Ian's special situation? What is kinesthesia made up of? In the previous chapter, we associated the term with certain combinations of sensations that go with the sense of the body's movements. Ian's success shows surprisingly that we can control our movements through vision even when other sensory feedback is missing. But it comes at a high price.

DISTINGUISHING MECHANICAL
FROM VISUAL KINESTHESIA

In their 1973 paper, "The Autonomy of Visual Kineasthesis," University of Edinburgh perception scientists J. R. Lishman and David Lee drew a distinction between two aspects of kinesthesia: mechanical and visual. We might assume that mechanical kinesthesia—or the information from the sensory receptors in the joints and soft tissue—is primary. However, Lishman and Lee used the term *visual kinesthesia* to emphasize the significance of this second way we have to find ourselves. To demonstrate the independence of the two kinds of kinesthesia, the researchers conducted the following experiments.

In the first test in the experiment, subjects were asked to walk down a dark corridor, while the researchers projected a landscape moving past them on the walls. The subjects reported that they were moving forward.

In the second test, the subjects were likewise in a dark corridor, and they saw a landscape projected on the walls moving past them as they walked forward; they reported that they were moving forward, just like in the first test. But in this second test, at a certain moment as the subjects continued to walk forward, the researchers reversed the film: the projected landscape was now moving in the same direction as the subjects. Even though the subjects were still actually walking forward, this time they reported moving backwards. Their movements had not changed, but their perception aligned with their visual experience of the landscape moving forward, not the mechanical information they were still receiving from the receptors in their tissue. Visual kinesthesia won over mechanical kinesthesia, and they experienced an illusion of walking backwards. You may have felt a version of this experience when sitting on a train in the station and the train next to you begins to move. If you are stationary, you may have a sense that you are moving backwards for a moment.

Lishman and Lee's study is an important example of how visual kinesthesia can dominate when there is a conflict between the visual information and the information coming from the receptors in our soft tissue and joints, the mechanical kinesthesia. In Ian's case, thanks to visual kinesthesia, he was able to use the information about his surroundings coming through his visual system to move, even without feeling anything of his own body.

Visual kinesthesia is powerful. For Ian, this was a constructive strategy, but for the rest of us, it's a double-edged sword. Vision can trump our sense of our body, and it is easy to fool. For instance, in Chapter Ten, when Sy looked in the mirror to find his good posture, the strategy had mixed results. He ended up looking good, but not finding good balance. Lishman and Lee's experiments show that visual information can take over, and we lose touch with the feeling of where we are. We can use vision skillfully, but in this visually dominated age, too often there is a deficit of attending to the other important sensory cues. This is often seen in the aging population: vision becomes the primary balancing mechanism while the sense reception through the feet diminishes, leading to a decrease in toe strength and an increased risk of falls (Mickle *et al.*, 2009; Yeh *et al.*, 2014).

TRY THIS

On the simplest level, understanding these two forms of kinesthesia can redirect what we imagine we are exercising while exercising. For example:

- We may want to turn away from the mirror, away from visual input, while we are moving.
- We may want to tune up mechanical kinesthesia, closing our eyes in simple, safe movements, to tune in to the streams of information other than vision that are available to us.
- We may want to use eye movements, changing the focal length looking out into the distance and following our hands with our eyes, out to the horizon and back in towards the body, in order to exercise the way we use our eyes to orient.

Including new terms, new images, new understanding of what is involved in movement, how visual and mechanical kinesthesia work autonomously and together, can help expand our personal movement practices in a myriad of ways.

EXPANDING THE CONCEPT OF PROPRIOCEPTION

The details of Ian's story show us that the terms "proprioception" and "kinesthesia" are too simple to describe body awareness and movement capacity. Ian lost his proprioceptors, but he was able to move by using the frame of reference the world provides. Moving isn't just about sensing ourselves from the inside: to move, we also use the world we sense around us.

In his 1978 article, "The Functions of Vision," Lee poses the question: how do we (human beings) situate ourselves in the environment (1978, p.160)? Following Gibson, Lee orients his question to emphasize the relationship with the environment, changing the frame of the inquiry. The question is not answered by something inside alone, but by an interaction between our perceptual systems and the information available in our surroundings. Remember the robotics researchers' formulation: to consider embodiment, they look at the "coupling between brain, body and environment" (Pfeifer and Bongard, 2007, p.20). The term "body awareness" doesn't remind us that we are embedded in an environment, so researchers like Lee found other terms to use.

Lee distinguishes three kinds of information that we gather to situate ourselves in the environment:

- Proprioceptive information is "about the positions and movements of the parts of the body relative to the body—the relation of body parts."
- Exteroceptive information is about the layout of the environment and about external objects and events.[1] Exteroceptive information is not limited to vision, but can include other senses, such as the sounds, smells, and touch of our surroundings.
- Lee adds a third dimension he calls "ex-proprioception," which he defines as using the environment as the frame of reference to obtain information about the body itself or part of it: "the obtaining of information about the position, orientation or movement of the body as a whole, or part of the body, relative to the environment" (Lee, 1978, p. 160).

For Ian, the ex-proprioceptive information supplied by vision was the key to his rehabilitation. Vision allowed him to find himself relative to his environment even though he couldn't feel his body. He still had the ex-proprioceptive information from his vestibular system, and he could substitute ex-proprioceptive visual information for the loss of his joint receptors. As time went on, he found that he could even drive: controlling a car primarily requires using ex-proprioceptive information; our view of the world *outside* gives us the feedback we need about where we are and how fast the car is going.

Applied to ourselves, Lee says that with these three kinds of information, we can accomplish any activity. Let's use tennis as an example. To plan an act in the world, we use exteroceptive information: I need to see where the net is—the layout of the external environment—if I want to hit the tennis ball over it. To control the act in process, we use proprioceptive/kinesthetic information. My proprioceptors help me set the proper muscle tone to hold and swing the racquet. I use ex-proprioceptive information in both circumstances—planning and action. Ex-proprioception helps me to keep my orientation in gravity and to situate myself relative to the net and the tennis court and sky around me. Our visual pathways can provide all three types of information: proprioceptive, exteroceptive, and ex-proprioceptive.

PRACTICAL APPLICATIONS

Do we need so many terms? What does the idea of ex-proprioception add for those of us who, unlike Ian, have intact proprioception and kinesthesia?

Coaches can use Gibson and Lee's framework to optimize athletic performance (Gray, 2024). The key to becoming a better mover is, as Hubert liked to say, "to choose the good information," which will depend on the context. Proprioceptive training, such as slow shifting of weight from one foot to the other that we find in tai chi practice, for example, can enable us to perceive an imbalance: I might not have noticed feeling less supported when shifting onto my left leg. The slow practice will allow me to pay attention to receiving information about the floor and my balance point through my left foot, priming a useful neurological pathway. But in the moment of action, the information from the environment about where I am situated—ex-proprioception—is more important and immediate. Following Gibson, each one of these ways of situating ourselves can be developed so that we become more skillful—able to adapt comfortably to many situations.

Understanding ex-proprioception can also help us build a more reliable body on an emotional level. For example, let's say I am walking in a room in which my friend is sitting in a chair. I might not be paying attention to the feeling of my body moving, but visually I can tell that I moved relative to them. In this case, I am using my friend as a reference point for orientation. Why is this a problem? Because that person can move. If I am depending on something (someone) that can move for my own balance, I must constantly adjust in response to that person. It's not hard to see that this strategy—using something that can change as a source of stability—might lead to hyper-vigilance. It may not be the most dependable form of ex-proprioceptive information. Understanding this empowers me to choose a better strategy.

Tuning ex-proprioception

In addition, we can tune ex-proprioception. As Edward Reed points out in his seminal paper, "An Outline of a Theory of Action Systems," "A *posture* is an orientation of the animal with respect to its environment" (1982, p.118). How would I go about tuning ex-proprioception?

Instead of using the stressful visual reference described above, I can practice orienting through my sense of weight to feel the ground and my sense of the surrounding space/sky to access vestibular information as we explored in Chapter Eight. These are more stable features of the environment and provide better information about general orientation. Choosing ground and sky allows me to situate myself relative to these more permanent references and leaves me with comfortable options whether the Other stays still, comes closer, or leaves the room.

Without the concept and language to describe subtle differences, would we even think that we can change our state of being or increase our sense of security by simply shifting our attention to a more constructive element of the environment? Instead of overusing a visual impression of the person in front of me to help me maintain balance, choosing them as my frame of reference, I can choose the chair I am sitting on or the floor under my feet, change my gaze to shift the vanishing point to go beyond the person in front of me, or, as we will go into later (Chapter Fifteen), the sense of the space behind and above me.

In another example of the practical use of these concepts, Hubert used Lee's framework as an innovative approach to movement analysis in his work with breast cancer patients at the National Cancer Institute in Milan, Italy. The patients had unexpected movement deficits—in particular, in arm swing—with no corresponding lack of muscle strength. Instead, they were missing the orientation provided by ex-proprioception that helps us coordinate action. Exteroception is a way of inhabiting the space around us; this too was impacted by the breast cancer diagnosis. (I will go into detail about this research in Chapter Sixteen.) The way we perceive the world around us is literally shaping us.

Perception has many layers. Distinctions allow us to describe our embodiment more clearly and give us something practical. More ways to orient give us more options to be safe and secure while other elements change. We are now going to go back to our original terms "body image" and "body schema" to discover what new possibilities they will open for us.

REVISITING BODY IMAGE AND BODY SCHEMA

One way to describe Ian's experience is to say that he lost the information flow that allowed the movement system to form an adequate body schema, an internal sense of where he was in space, and that he was able to find a way to move again primarily thanks to his body image, his conscious ability to see himself, and the ex-proprioceptive power of vision.

Connecting body image and schema to What and Where pathways

Another perspective on body image and body schema comes from Jacques Paillard, a pioneering French neurophysiologist who studied our sense of movement. Paillard linked body image and body schema with the two visual pathways in the brain, What (ventral) and Where (dorsal) (Chapter Three). He suggests that "the location of body parts in a *body schema* (a 'where' problem in the body space) could be differently processed in the CNS [central nervous system] than the perceptual identification of the body features in a *body image* (a 'what' problem)" (Paillard, 1999, p.198). Faced with skepticism from fellow neurologists, Paillard wanted to preserve the concept of body schema because it bridges neurophysiology and psychology, differentiating the sensorimotor aspect of experience from the cognitive. The What pathway is linked to language centers, allowing us to identify and name things cognitively. The Where pathway, the sensorimotor domain, works first and faster, and helps us navigate our environment. As we saw in Chapter Three, using the Where pathway keeps us in touch with our whereabouts more directly, picking up on shape and movement. Ian's experience is thus the opposite of the blindsight patients': having lost the Where pathway, he used his What pathway to move his body. In general, we are more identified with the "what," the cognitive aspect of self, than we are with what our body schema does for us. Ian Waterman once again provides a stark example of what would be required for any of us to move without the contributions of the Where system.

For Ian to move, he had to take over the subconscious processes that become the body schema, deconstruct the enormous number of individual sub-movements and compensations, and do each part through deliberate will. Without proprioceptive information, when he began to try to walk again, he had to figure out how to plan for balance changes. Ian learned the hard way, through falling, that every movement had to be preceded by managing his center of gravity. Without sensation, he had to do all this through careful planning and intention, remembering each aspect of each step. Like the robotics engineers in Part I, before his illness, Ian had no idea what the body schema was doing for him. After his illness, using planning and vision, his conscious mind (body image) was able to make up for the body schema's missing information. But it was a colossal effort.

As he learned a new way to walk, Ian had to stand with his feet far apart to maintain his balance. He couldn't let his knees bend or his legs would collapse. His entire body became very stiff when he stood or walked. To move his foot forward without dragging it, he lifted it high to the side and then dropped it hard on his heel. His movements were jerky, tense, and slow, as if he were a wooden puppet controlled by a beginner. The whole process was utterly exhausting

In one video, Ian is seen walking at a good clip down the street. But there is something unusual about the way he walks: he leads with his feet and looks at them. He explains:

> I have to scan the path ahead, not immediately in front of my feet but probably about six or eight feet ahead. I'm planning all the time exactly what's coming up. I've got to be aware of where I am going to place my feet so that I don't compromise myself. (BBC Horizon, 1998, 13:22–13:52; Cole, 1995, pp.61–62)

He can't afford to be distracted.

Ian's example brings home to us just how much of the process of movement happens beneath the surface, based in perceptual processes we take for granted—what we are here calling the body schema. His apparent recovery of function hid the prodigious acts of memory and concentration he engaged in to move at all. To this day, Ian's every act must be thought through, practiced, and controlled, requiring enormous attention. Every day is a marathon, a sustained effort for each and every step.

Kinetic melody

Movement has a flow to it that has been likened to music, the kinetic melodies we observed previously with Laney and Brendan (Chapter Seven). Although each person has a unique signature, there is a smooth flow for most of us that is missing for Ian. It may be possible to substitute ex-proprioceptive information for kinesthetic awareness, but Ian's story shows us the difficulty of moving from an external image. Not only is it an enormous effort to move with only visual kinesthesia, but it is also a huge loss. The music of movement can't be replaced by deliberate action.

Ian's experience reminds us of the underpinnings of our movements, the need for balance, and the degree to which the capacity to form some kind of body schema, upon which our movements depend, is informed by kinesthetic information rather than by conscious muscular control. Seen from this perspective, what is the use of all the injunctions to stand up straight and pull our shoulders back or our stomachs in for good posture? The most important work happens *before* we act, through our choice of perceptual information to prepare the movement—pre-movement.

BODY IMAGE AND SCHEMA IN PRACTICE

Body image, in Head and Holmes' (1911) sense of a conscious representation of our body, is a mixed blessing. It's inevitable that we develop an image of what we look like. It may be conscious, but that doesn't mean it's accurate, efficient, or even well suited to the job of organizing movement. Ian used conscious control in a positive way to manage his unusual circumstances, but for most of us, deliberate muscular control, watching ourselves in a mirror, or imagining how we look to someone else will not lead to flow in movement, to a beautiful kinetic melody.

How does the body schema/body image distinction contribute to our understanding and practice of movement? In 1974, Tim Gallwey first published *The Inner Game of Tennis, The Classic Guide to the Mental Side of Peak Performance.* The inner game, Gallwey wrote, is played within our own minds between Self 1, the inner critic, whose running commentary of negative remarks we hear in our heads when trying something new, and Self 2 who just learns by doing.

You can see clips of Gallwey from years ago on YouTube (TheCoach, 2012). In the video, Gallwey recruits a complete novice to tennis, a woman who has never before held a racket. His instructions are very simple: he has her watch him hit the ball with a partner and tells her to say "bounce" exactly when the ball hits the court and "hit" when he hits the ball. At first, she just watches him and says the words as the ball bounces, and he hits the ball with a partner. Then he has her say the words as the ball is hit towards her but tells her not to worry about hitting the ball. And finally, when she is ready, she hits the ball as she says the words. To her own surprise, with this simple set of cues she is able to begin to return the volleys with no trouble.

Gallwey's explanation is that his cues distract Self 1 from its litany of negativity and also keep its attention from wandering, but it's clear that he is asking for sensory cues—the rhythm and timing of saying the words, listening to the sound the ball makes against the racket, the dance of the serve—all his cues are actually very effective ways to speak to the body schema. Like Hubert, he is directing the novice's attention to useful information for the movement system. Not a word about body parts, where her hand or feet should be, nothing about her own body, how she should stand—at all!

Without the concept of body schema, the importance of addressing it in movement education gets lost, and people go on to this day trying to teach movement by telling people where to put their body parts—engaging the body image in a less effective strategy for movement. Over the past 50 years, without the words to describe the body schema, *The Inner Game* evolved to be an executive coaching strategy focused on the inner critic. Yet as a somatic practice, we find that helping our sense of orientation, working with the body schema directly, contributes to building a reliable body and to our sense of emotional security. It's not all in our heads!

Through Ian's story told in Chapters Ten and Eleven, it's clear that the body image/schema doesn't tell the whole story of body awareness, but it can be a very handy distinction for movement teachers. By understanding the less conscious aspects of movement, we can begin to partner with our movement system.

Neuroscientists such as Paillard, philosophers such as Gallagher, and medical doctors like Cole are all in agreement that the movement system perceives the world through different streams of information, not as a seamless flow. From these different streams of information, we construct a view, associate meaning and memories, and call it reality. Understanding how movement processes work, as we have been exploring throughout this chapter, allows us to become more discerning about what's wrong and how to help. We can partner with the body schema by guiding our perceptual choices instead of by controlling our muscular system. The next section shows how we would apply this framework to refine balance and develop our ability to manage our instability.

TRIANGLE OF BALANCE

In "The Functions of Vision," Lee explores the information we need to control balance. We use ex-proprioceptive information about where we are (orientation) and how we are moving relative to the environment so that the muscles can properly adapt to changing circumstances. We keep in touch with the environment through our senses through: "1) inertial contact through the vestibular system; 2) physical contact through the feet; and 3) optical contact through the eye" (Lee, 1978, p.161). Lee classifies all three elements as ex-proprioception because balance is accomplished in relation to an environment. These three information sources—the inner ear, the receptors in the feet, and the role of vision—make up what Hubert called the "triangle of balance" (or "posture" in the sense of what remains the same while other aspects change; what we do to not fall down).

These terms give us a range of options to work with, for ourselves or as practitioners working with others. As Gibson said, perception is a skill that we can work with. We can use a variety of sources of information instead of getting stuck in one channel. To the goal of building muscular strength, we can add developing adaptable perceptual strategies. When Hubert would say, "We are practicing choosing the good information," he meant the good information for each one of us, at this moment, in this context. Freshly.

> ### TRY THIS ✓
> To this day, I find the triangle of balance concept a useful framework for my own movement practice. What information am I tuning in to, to organize balance and orientation? Eyes, inner ear (the vestibular system), and the sensory receptors of each foot are the important sources for balance. How am I using each of these?
>
> In class, Hubert would have us start an embodiment by letting go from a standing position, letting go of whatever we are doing

to stay upright, as I did with Sy. This brings me to hang down a little, to release any holding in my shoulders and back. From this new posture, new information is available. I might feel the ground through the soles of my feet more—that is common. Or I notice the way one leg takes more weight than the other.

Then, for example, we would use the image of the snake rising, with coils still on the ground (a variation of the yoga asana Cobra) to trigger activity in the vestibular system, to wake up the inner ear. Remember from Chapter Eight how the vestibular system participates in the multisensory integration that leads to the world appearing coherent.

To use this idea in movement, Hubert encouraged us to use other senses to trigger the return to the initial upright position: we could listen to the sounds around us, allowing the auditory system to help us find our way to upright and oriented.

We could get a whiff of scent in the air, using the olfactory system, which can be a powerful aid to orientation.

We could come up putting our attention on the way the air feels on the skin of our face, or imagining ourselves in safe waters, as if we could feel the water on the skin all over the body.

We could let focal vision relax in favor of peripheral—or occasionally to alternate focal and peripheral vision—to get the eyes out of their patterned use.

Activating any of these sensory streams is a way to stimulate vestibular function, to trigger the body schema's capacity to help with orientation. We were actively choosing to vary the information sources: visual, vestibular, and proprioceptive through the foot's contact with the ground.

These suggestions also turned our attention away from standing up the usual way, from a familiar effort leading to a familiar end result. Instead, we were learning and practicing paying attention to the perceptual information available at the moment.

Hubert understood that perception is selective,[2] that our habits are based in inadvertently firing the same neurons over and over. But new information is always available, and Hubert's instructions encouraged us to select new pathways each time. *Could I keep the feeling of the ground, of soft feet, that I found when I let go, as I begin to come up? As I engage my eyes?*

Part of embodiment is to practice perceptual skills: to deliberately choose a different information source than our habitual one. By understanding the role and dimensions of the perceptual processes that inform us about the world, we can learn to change troublesome movement patterns by starting with perception, before we move, and using Hubert's formula: 50 percent body, 50 percent world.

As we have seen, below the level of consciousness each of us uses different streams of information to keep ourselves oriented. Below the level of consciousness, micro-adjustments are triggered to maintain posture and manage weight shift based on predictions derived from past experience. When we exercise, for example, we may think of our squats as a workout for quads or glutes or hamstrings, but simultaneously, subconsciously, many other muscles participate in each movement to keep us from falling over. Pre-movements are *anticipatory* by necessity. The anticipatory—that is, predictive—nature of movement planning reveals an important aspect of how our habits work for us and sometimes against us (Gurfinkel, 1994). Prediction must be based on past experience, on memory; it is a path we have traveled before. The anticipatory gesture may happen below the level of consciousness, but its impact is accessible. When we know where to put our attention, our consciousness can contribute to developing options for the body schema, leading to a wide range of strategies to help us navigate each situation.

CHAPTER TWELVE

Meeting the World

Jonathan Cole's gripping account of Ian's story reveals the importance of kinesthesia and its complexity. Without the information usually supplied by receptors about position and movement, only Ian's remarkable will enabled him to reclaim some physical capacities—standing, walking, studying, and working—by using visual information. Three years after the onset of his illness, Ian was well enough to attend school and eventually took a job in an office, but he vividly described the challenges of his situation. Sometimes he would wake to feel a hand on his face and not know to whom it belonged. Until he realized it was his own hand, the experience was momentarily terrifying (Cole, 1995, p.85). It is so hard for us to imagine what this experience would be like!

Apart from the difference in the way he walks, Ian looks like the rest of us, so people around him do not necessarily understand how he moves through the world differently than they do. Because he doesn't get sensory feedback, a windy day or simply being touched can be destabilizing. When he goes to a bar, for example, he sits with his back against something because being slapped on the back or bumped would knock him over. Like the first biped robots, he can be thrown off balance by just picking up a squash in the supermarket. We cannot truly imagine the kind of vigilance required when a gust of wind or a well-intentioned pat on the back can knock you over! Conversely, Ian's experience vividly brings home to us how each moment we are keeping in touch with our world through kinesthetic information.

Without an example such as Ian's, it would be hard to recognize the magnitude of the signals we are continually processing that allow us to stay in touch with our surroundings. The world tells us where we are moment to moment through whatever we are touching or what touches us, a tactile version of ex-proprioceptive information (the way we find ourselves from the outside in). So much depends on the sensory conversation that is going on between us and our changing environment!

It was hard for Ian to express what he felt in part because we don't have words to describe or familiarity with what our kinesthetic sense does for us. The processes that go into body schema are not fully understood and are mostly ignored in favor of willful activity. Ian's story shows us the enormous mechanical job that is required to fill the kinesthetic void that the body schema—the model of movement updated each moment—does for us. But Ian's loss was more than mechanical: the kinesthetic sense that keeps us in touch with our surroundings also participates in our sense of orientation and our sense of security.

SENSE OF SELF, SENSE OF SECURITY

In one study, the doctors wanted to observe Ian's brain activity through an MRI scanner. For the test, Ian had to lie still on his back, unable to see his body. The MRI showed activation in the part of his brain that looks for feedback, but what Ian felt was extreme anxiety.[1]

Ian's experience in the MRI machine reminds us that the feedback our system gets from our proprioceptors through contact with our surroundings can keep us oriented, acting as a kind of reassurance. While kinesthesia, proprioception, orientation, and perception may seem like purely physiological issues, they are deeply tied to our sense of safety and well-being.

Usually, "proprioception" is used as a catch-all for "perception or awareness of the position and movement of the body." But now you can see the beautiful complexity covered over by this term. In the context of how we know where we are, how we keep our balance, there is an inherent relationship with where we are, an ongoing connection.

When Ian's doctor, Jonathan Cole, chose to use the term "kinesthesia" for the sixth sense, he may have been sensitive to the implications. Proprioception and kinesthesia carry different connotations. *Proprio* means self, so what is implied is that body awareness is of "self," whereas *kine* means to move, and *aesthis* is sensation—the feeling of moving. Kinesthesia does not specify a subject, but rather offers an invitation into relationship with the surroundings, a meeting.

HOW WE MEET THE WORLD

How we meet the world is an important dimension in practice, whether we are working with our own movement system or with someone else's. One September, at a workshop in a Spanish beach town south of Cadiz, Hubert recounted the roots of his insight on this topic (Cadiz workshop, 2013). Years before, he had taken a workshop with Dominique Dupuy, the French dancer and choreographer. Dupuy had the students hold a stick as part of a movement practice. Hubert thought he was following Dupuy's instructions, but as Dupuy passed by, he said to Hubert, "Where you are is not where it is." In a flash, Hubert understood what was missing in his movement: the quality of contact with the stick.

In the previous chapters, we have explored the different sources of perceptual information we use to support active movement. The story Hubert told at that workshop invited us to explore the question from the other side: what are the movements that serve perception? In the example of holding a stick, tiny changes in the muscles in the palm and hand, supported by small changes in the arm and in the whole body in relation to breath and to stability, are all movements that shape the quality of contact—with the stick, or the floor, or another person.

Movements in service of perception are not grand, sweeping gestures. If we want to feel something, to perceive something, smaller movements are required: we run our fingers over a surface, or we make micro-adjustments with our head to see more clearly. Some of these are micro-movements, barely visible from outside.

When I take my dog Bodhi for a walk, I have a chance to observe the delicate movements she makes in service of her sense of smell. Her whole body orients as she senses something that compels her attention. As she sniffs, she might tilt her head back to pick up a scent on the breeze, or bury her nose in the yard's grass, or circle the fire hydrant, nose to the ground, to find out who else has been there. The micro-movements help her follow the swirls and waves of the molecules that make up the bouquet of odors and direct them into the back of her snout where she can find out more about them.[2] Like Bodhi, subtle movements allow us to take in more information about what we are smelling, seeing, hearing, or touching. And just like the pre-movements of orientation we considered in previous chapters, they are shaping what can be perceived.

Hubert used the term *haptos* to describe these movements that support perceiving and meeting objects and the world. Haptic capacity was

another dimension of in-touchness that Ian lost. Ian described the difficulty of learning to handle an egg—to gauge how much pressure would
prevent the egg from slipping from his fingers but not break the shell.
This movement capacity was also a problem for some early robots. They
might very impressively serve coffee, or they might crush the cup instead.
The mundane act of handling an egg or a cup requires a complex combination of perception and action, of anticipation and feedback from the
present moment. Although for most of us handling objects usually takes
place without much thought, it is actually a complex act of coordination.

"Why am I choosing to use this special word?" Hubert asked. "We
already have a lot of words: mechanoreceptors, sensitivity of the feet,
kinesthesia, proprioception, et cetera. So why use a different word like
haptic?" Hubert explained that while mechanoreceptors brought sensory
information, and muscle spindles brought kinesthetic information, we
would use the term "haptic" to describe a special motor skill that was not
for the purpose of moving, but instead to help orient the sensory organs
(Cadiz workshop, 2013). Haptic in this sense describes the small motor
acts that shape the contact of our hands with the stick when we hold it,
or our feet with the floor—the moment of meeting. Using the term *haptos*
helped us to notice that there were several dimensions in the process we
call "touch."

In the early 1900s, Gestalt philosophers described touch as made up
of two distinct actions: "touch" described the more passive aspect and
"kinesthesia" described the active, seeking, dimension (Grunwald, 2008).
Gibson and Paillard, among others, extended the idea to other senses.
(Gibson, 1966; Paillard, 1999). Hubert was following this path as he introduced the term *haptos* to us: to help us explore the way we meet the world.
Without a term, this action of perception could be completely missed.
Hubert understood Dupuy's remark—"where it is"—to mean that the life
in the movement, the newness, the now-ness, was in the meeting of the
hand and the stick.

Hubert began to notice this quality of contact in his practice with
clients (personal communication, December 13, 2019). One patient had
developed pain in his right foot when he walked. The examination showed
no obvious structural problem and neither motor nor neurological issues.
When the patient was asked to move his foot voluntarily, he could do it.
With the patient lying on the table, Hubert asked him to push against
Hubert's hand, using one foot and then the other. Hubert perceived a surprising difference between the action of the two feet. From the left foot,

there was strong contact, a definitive push. In contrast. as the right foot met Hubert's palm, the patient reported having no feeling of contact. His right side seemed almost inert. The problem manifested only in contact with a surface (e.g., Hubert's hand, or the ground in walking). The motor inhibition only arose in the moment of contact, when the patient had to meet the world. The quality of contact of Hubert's patient with the floor led to his discomfort. Hubert coined the term "haptic dissociation" to describe the problem he observed in his client. He noticed that medical tests would miss the issue: the touch capacity is present; the motor capacity is intact. But the two capacities are not working together. This is why he came to give it a special name. The "lesion" he noticed in his patient was in the haptic system. *Haptos* refers to the movements which magnify and orient our sensory activity.

> The movement of the body, which is at the service of my eyes, or at the service of my inner ear, or at the service of my sense of touch of feet and hands, this particular movement is "haptic." For me to see you, the muscles of my body have to participate.

He said: "This differs from *motricité* [motor skill] to move; it's a *motricité* to help my eyes, to help my capacity of touch, to help my capacity to hear, to work together." Originally, haptic only applied to touch, but after Gibson and others, Hubert extended the notion to vision and to audition.

Hubert adopted the term "haptic dissociation" to describe the problem he observed in his client. He found that the dissociation came before orienting; it was in the movement of the body to explore the world. In situations of physical or emotional trauma, what is often lost is exactly this in-touchness, the haptic capacity, the movements that support feeling and perceiving. In meeting the world, we can accept the touch, or we can reject it. Hubert introduced a distinction between two ways haptic capacity can function in ourselves and the people we work with: either with an openness to exploration or to establish a protective or defensive separation in our encounter with the world. Both of these stances use the same mechanism. Haptic dissociation gives us a pathway to work with some post-traumatic situations, by slowly re-establishing the ongoing movements of connection that keep us in touch.

Hubert's use of the terms *haptos* and "haptic capacity" is particular to him and to the context of working with patients and students to change movement abilities. In scientific literature, the term "haptic" is used to

refer to the sense of touch without bringing out the special motor function required.

Long before adopting the term, Hubert had encountered perplexing
situations in clinical settings. One example he recounted to me was of an
electrician who was fixing an alarm system when the alarm went off right
in his ear. From that time on, the electrician experienced deafness, but
mysteriously the doctors could not find any physiological problem with
his hearing. Understanding the problem through the phenomenological
lens, Hubert realized that his patient was in a protective defense against
sounds and successfully worked with the electrician to slowly reopen the
capacity to open to the sounds around him.

Hubert's idea of *haptos* and my experiences working with him using
the concept (see Introduction/*Stick work* and Chapter Eight/*Sun salute*),
helped me understand that perception is not a passive process. In just the
action of touching the stick I am going to pick up, there is already complex
coordination. Not only am I preparing a movement of picking up the
stick, which requires balancing, but also at that moment I am practicing
a way of contacting, coordinating small muscles that create a particular
quality of touch. *Haptos* is another dimension of pre-movement. To affect
this level takes time and willingness not to know, to give the sensations
of this moment a chance to come in, to meet anew. Remember the 200
milliseconds required for an impression to come to consciousness (Chapter 3). Giving that time to receive before acting—short as it is—allows
this moment to come to my senses rather than operating entirely on
previous programming. This is what changes our brain's map. Through
his approach, Hubert was teaching us to allow a new coordination, a new
meeting that would feed fresh information to the somatosensory cortex
and thus provide a new ground for action.

ANTICIPATION: EVOLUTIONARY
ADVANTAGE OR DRAWBACK?

Going back to Ian's description of the challenge of picking up an egg in
the supermarket: without the immediate feedback from his fingers about
what they were touching, vision was not enough to supply information
about the exact amount of tension needed so he wouldn't drop the egg
but would not break the fragile shell either.

The neuroscientist Alain Berthoz sums up Ian's difficulty calibrating the pressure of his fingers on an eggshell with only vision in a simple phrase: how not to crush a raspberry (Berthoz, 2009/2012, p.86). Berthoz has written extensively about the underpinnings of the haptic sense. His definition is the usual one: the sense of touch or perception through touch.

> In feeling an object to test its shape or gauge its weight, or in caressing a person we desire, we not only call into play the tactile sense through the many receptors situated in and under the skin. We also activate proprio-ceptive (sense of the body) sensors situated in the muscles and joints, and we associate that activity with a sense of muscular effort. This complex ensemble, which requires elaborate multisensory integration, is what we call the haptic sense. (Berthoz, 2009/2012, pp.84–85)

Berthoz describes what the movement system is up to in what seems like a simple act. Below the level of consciousness, in preparing to move, preparing to touch, we are recalling previously learned strategies from memory. When you pick something up, you—but perhaps not the "you" that you identify with—make decisions based on past perceptual and movement experience. How heavy the book is, previous raspberries you have interacted with, for example—these memories will be evoked and, inevitably, anticipation will come into play when we move, touch, and interact.

Our repertoire of experience is based on several layers. Some move-ments seem to be hardwired, inherited from our ancestors' evolution in relationship with their environment. We also make assumptions based on our own past experience about the weight of the object we are going to pick up and about how fragile and how easily crushed or broken an object is. Neuroscientists call this an internal model: we have an internal model of how easily crushed the raspberry will be. This model is based on memories starting from our earliest experiences, ones we may not remember consciously. Yet we are using these memories, building on our experience base from our first year or two to predict—to plan ahead with lightning speed—as we pick up today's raspberry.

As we reach for the berry, our movement system anticipates based on past experience to set the tone of the muscles used for grasping it. In addi-tion, at the moment of contact, new information about this particular rasp-berry—how it feels now—is available. Anticipation is but one part; what allows the egg to be picked up or the raspberry not be crushed is a moment of perceiving the particular egg or raspberry in the present. When we move our fingers around a ball, we get a sense of the ball's shape, size, weight, texture, et cetera, from our skin but also from our movements, from the kinesthetic motor activity that Hubert calls haptic activity.

Even without touch, we can perceive the form of an object "without any proprioceptive, kinesthetic, or motor information" (Berthoz, 2009/2012, p.87). Vision on its own can convey very physical information. Berthoz describes an experiment performed by computer scientist Anatole Lécuyer in which viewers observed an image of a virtual piston pressing on a spring on a computer screen. Participants could use the computer mouse to push down the piston in the image; as long as the image on the screen mirrored the spring slowing down, as the person would expect, they reported feeling the force of the piston's operation on the mouse. Lécuyer called this illusion of force "pseudo-haptic illusion" in which "a single piece of visual information induces the illusion of a force applied to the hand" (Berthoz, 2009/2012, p.87). In this way, vision can substitute to some extent for proprioception, as Ian also discovered. Berthoz elegantly paraphrases Merleau-Ponty: "vision is the brain's way of touching" (Berthoz, 2009/2012, p.87; Merleau-Ponty, 1964, p.175).

How does all this apply to our everyday movements?

Perception is a combination of past and present. Anticipation—the history of how we move—is necessary for us to function. We have to move forward in part based on memory and prediction. For example, our movement system shapes our hand differently, in anticipation, depending on what we are about to pick up. But there is also the perception that comes from the present moment, when we meet the raspberry and have a chance to finely modulate just how much pressure we need to use to pick up this particular raspberry. This moment. This meeting. This exchange. Not from memory.

EMBODIMENT AND PLASTICITY

What Hubert called haptic dissociation was a protective gesture—not quite letting in the moment. By calling attention to this action, and applying a particular name, Hubert brought out a dimension of practice that is easily missed. In the context of exercising, everyday activities, or meeting each other, we may not realize how we are engaging or disengaging or how to get back in touch.

TRY THIS ✅

Haptic activity

To evoke a lived experience of the concept of *haptos*, Hubert would have us lie on the floor, knees bent, feet against the wall. "Let the wall become soft, let the feet melt into a wall that is like butter," he would suggest, instead of telling us to push the wall. Subtle movements of my legs and feet let me feel that the wall was touching me, that the wall was soft. That starting point would trigger better core stabilization than any deliberate contraction of particular muscles, as we found ourselves moving away from the wall without the tension of our usual way of pushing.

We can have a new meeting, this moment. That's the quality of being in touch—touching and being touched—that Merleau-Ponty refers to as an intertwining—where each sense can be both active (touching) and receptive (touched) (Bernard, 2019). It's what I experienced working with the stick—what Hubert named *haptos* or haptic capacity. It is a movement, it is imagination, it is a perception in the moment. It's an alternative to directing body parts through voluntary contraction (so common in movement classes of all kinds). Instead, movement practices working with haptic capacity could help us to get back in touch literally and allow us time (those 200 milliseconds!) for a new perception, a different starting point for the movement. This is a key element in changing our movement patterns for the better.

Our movement capacity affects our sense of self and our sense of connection. Throughout Part III, we have been exploring what terms we can use to work more effectively with our own movement system. What can we learn from Ian's experience about how to teach movement or try to change our own or someone else's movement pattern? Although we usually don't have to think about it, having a more complex set of terms helps us have better access to the complex phenomenon of embodiment.

How do we use the terms "body schema" and "plasticity" in relation to movement practice? Body schema is a provisional concept that represents a function that is taking place in multiple locations; it's a system, rather than an organ or a specific place in the brain. Ian's initial shock of not feeling the usual channels of sensory information and the subsequent discovery of other channels that allowed him to locate himself are examples of neuroplasticity—the network of nerve cells throughout the body can change its tuning. At first, with the primary channel lost, Ian felt that he had entirely lost a sense of where his body was. But over time, he became aware of other channels—slower input, but still valuable information.

Head and Holmes' original definitions in which body schema is unconscious and body image is conscious break down—is Ian using body image to move or did he develop a new body schema? But this is not what matters. The time spent imagining what would be lost if we didn't have kinesthesia lets us access a kaleidoscope of perceptual processes with which we can meet the world.

The capacity for changing our tuning tells us something about the "perceptual body" that we all share with Ian. The nervous system is plastic: it changes according to what we pay attention to. Norman Doidge, author of *The Brain that Changes Itself* (2007), describes neuroplasticity as the brain's capacity to change its structure and function depending on what it does. When we are sensing and perceiving, what we react to will rewire our brains. Our actions, and even what we think and imagine, all change the structure of the brain.

Not just the brain in our heads, but the whole network of neurons is "livewired," to use David Eagleman's expression (2020). Each moment, our choices shape our wiring. As Ian's example shows us, we have to feel or perceive in order to move, and the way we go about it each moment—the channels we tune to—is shaping our whole system. Perceiving and moving create a feedback loop: perceiving allows us to move, and moving—the sensations registered from the movement—shapes our sensory maps.

Hubert introduced us to Michael Merzenich's research on the somatosensory cortex (part of the cerebral cortex) in the early 1990s, when brain plasticity was just beginning to be recognized by the scientific community. Merzenich challenged a then-primary assumption about brain organization: that the brain's map of the body is hardwired, unchanging (as cited in Doidge, 2007). Until this research, which became more widely known in the early 2000s, the neuroscientific community believed cortical connections did not change in adulthood (Kandel, 2006, p.216).

In one experiment, researchers taped a monkey's fingers together for a couple of weeks. With fMRI, they were able to see that the area of the somatosensory cortex that represented the immobilized finger *disappeared*—after only two weeks—and was taken over by adjacent areas. Not moving caused changes in the brain's map. But once the fingers were free to move again, the representation returned after a couple of weeks. The monkey research showed that moving brings about feeling, and feeling modifies the brain's map (Allard *et al.*, 1991; Clark *et al.*, 1988).

In another experiment, the researchers trained a monkey to keep its finger on a rotating disc for ten seconds at a time at just the right pressure to get a reward. Over thousands of successes, the increased stimulation also modified the somatosensory cortex, enlarging the area of finger representation. This became evidence for a hypothesis about what underlies some chronic pain: with constant signaling, an area of representation in the somatosensory cortex can grow bigger (Doidge, 2015; Jenkins *et al.*, 1990).

Our muscles and connective tissues need variability, alternating loading and unloading to stay adaptable and healthy. Yet the very nature of neurons leads to repeating patterns that we have traveled before: the familiar path is usually faster, and therefore it's more likely that's the way we will go. Any perceptual habit that continues unconsciously puts us at risk: continually loading joints and soft tissue may eventually create a symptom. We can use neuroplasticity to keep us out of ruts. Neuroplasticity tells us that change is possible. Somatic movement work has the potential to renew rather than repeat. What is required of us is to first understand how movement works and then to bring consciousness to accessible aspects of the process.

When Hubert used an expression like "perception is acceleration," he meant that in bringing our attention to a particular feeling or sensation, we could amplify the incoming stream of information. To perceive is to make a choice, to select. Tuning in would amplify or accelerate the perception. We could choose what signals to pay attention to and the quality of our attention. This is the basis of movement work from Hubert's point of view. The brain/body relationship is not a simple, fixed phenomenon, and movement practices are also neurological practices. We can use them to reinforce what we have done before, or we can use them as an opportunity to enhance plasticity by changing our tuning, varying our pre-movement selection. Being open to the present is a very physical act.

CHAPTER THIRTEEN

Body Images

CLIENT STORY: BENJAMIN

Benjamin, a tall, good-looking man in his mid-50s, bearded, his long hair done up in a bun, arrived for his second session, saying, "My shoulder is no better; in fact, it got worse." He continued:

> Of course, that might be because I am doing squats for my back, and I decided to use three-pound weights. I did it two days in a row, and after that my arm felt really weak. But anyway, I'm wondering how much time I should devote to Rolfing before I see results because I am here to fix this shoulder, and I could use this money for dental work that I really need.

He looks down through his glasses at me from across the room, waiting for a response.

I listen and exhale. It's the 5:30 session, the last of a long day, on Thursday, almost the end of the week. We're in my office on the eighth floor of a building on Massachusetts Avenue in Cambridge, as the last light fades away.

When people are in pain, they have every reason to be impatient. Symptoms are insistent. Pain demands attention, and the mission—making the symptom go away—becomes all encompassing. He has had this problem for quite a while, several years in fact, and has already tried many things to address it. After many years in practice, I understand the difficulty. I reply, "I would probably give it about three sessions before I would make an assessment. I understand your dilemma." I go on:

> But on the other hand, if the problem was local, then chances are it would have gotten better with one of the other things you tried. PT would have

helped, or chiropractic. So, I imagine the reason you decided to try Rolfing is to take a different approach.

One of Dr. Rolf's favorite lines was: "Where you think it is—it ain't." I understand this saying to mean that when there is a symptom—as in this situation where there is pain or weakness down the arm—do not assume that the symptom's location is the *cause* of the problem. I find myself using that mantra regularly because symptoms are compelling but they can also be a distraction that prevents us from finding the root of the problem. After invoking Dr. Rolf for myself, I take a moment to observe Benjamin with my Rolfer's eyes, to see and feel simultaneously how he is organizing himself in gravity.

Looking at Benjamin, I see someone who is holding himself up, using effort to keep his good posture. I see the muscles working in his neck and shoulders, the slight tuck of his chin. When he moves or stands, I see-feel the underlying posture: holding on tightly in his hips, almost tucking them, so his back is flat (his spine has a flattened lumbar curve). With that kind of holding, the natural movement of the upper body would be to round forward, as if he were on his way to curling into a ball. But since that's not a good way to walk around, his upper body has to compensate and pull itself back into a semblance of uprightness.

To get a feeling for this posture, using the description above, try out that strategy for yourself.

The result of all these strategies was that his upper back, neck, and shoulders all lived in a state of tension.

I do want to help his symptom go away, but if the short-term, symptom approach was going to work, it would have done so already through the other approaches he has tried. Pausing a moment to let any defensiveness pass, I continue: "We are going to try a different approach." I explain that we are addressing the postural underpinnings that made his neck and shoulders—the thoracic outlet—tight, thus creating compression on the nerves in that area. "That compression," I told him, "is probably involved in your symptoms."

"Thanks, that's helpful," he says. "That's exactly what I wanted to hear."

I ask Benjamin to lie down on the table, and I begin to free the soft tissue around his feet and lower legs to open up the possibilities of sensation and movement through them. "Even though the symptom is in the shoulder," I say, "I'm going to start here to see if we can help your body find a way to rest more easily."

Lying there, he asks, "What should I be paying attention to inside when I am walking?" I am a little surprised at the question from out of the blue. "Inside?" I ask him. "It's interesting that you put it that way. Walking seems to be more about exploring your environment."

Interoception

Benjamin raises what seems like an innocuous question, but which covers something very important. "Feeling inside" is the colloquial term for interoception. Interoception gives us a sense of the ongoing physiological state of our body, a well of impressions, somewhat below the level of consciousness—sensations like pleasant/unpleasant, arousing/calming, that we may interpret and associate with an emotional state. There is a growing tendency in the somatic community, as well as in some forms of meditation, yoga, and psychotherapy, to emphasize inside feeling as if it were the same as body awareness. It's easy to assume that feelings are inside and that these inside feelings are the basis of movement. But it's not the whole story. As we have been exploring, body awareness is a complex perception that includes inside and outside. "Where am I?" is as important as "How am I?" Proprioception/kinesthesia and interoception are both important. There is some overlap between them, but they are by no means the same.

Tuning in to inside feelings on their own, without orientation and connection, can feel overwhelming, terrible! Paying attention to *where* we are connects us to our surroundings and to ourselves, using the ex-proprioceptive information described in Chapter Eleven. When we are moving, we locate ourselves in reference to the surrounding space. The information that guides our movement when we walk comes from outside of us as well. Ian's progress reminds us of this: losing part of his proprioception affected his normal movement abilities. But the fact that he can drive and the story of his reclaiming his ability to walk show that the "body inside" is not all that navigating the world requires. Finding our way requires a combination, a balance between the two domains—50 percent body and 50 percent world.

As I pause before responding to Benjamin's question, in the distance I hear the sounds of rush-hour traffic, honking, trucks rumbling. Inside the room, the rush of forced hot air is coming through the vent. The surroundings make themselves known.

Then I respond:

When you are walking, you can pay attention to letting the world come to you. The feeling of the floor or the ground, when you push off with the foot that is behind. That's one point of contact, and when you land, there's another. The rest is what's coming to you from the world. That's a good place to put your attention when you are walking.

"Oh," he says, "that seems overwhelming, to let the world in." He added, "I am very defended."

I notice his choice of terms. There is a lot behind simple word choices. It sounds as though, in Benjamin's experience, there was too much information coming from the world around him, and he didn't know how to organize himself in relation to what felt like an overwhelming onslaught. This uncomfortable feeling could be part of what drove his tendency to look "inside," and it suggests a skill that could be developed.

Organizing sensory input can be a very challenging task, whether for a newborn, a child, or an adult. With all the sensory information from outside and inside, it is easy to feel overwhelmed. How do we create a secure envelope, a sense of wholeness that can allow us to manage the range of sensory experience? How do we approach this challenge from a somatic perspective? How do we establish a sense of security?

Hubert's words come back to me: he would say we need "backing"—in the metaphorical sense. Not a literal back, but to be well oriented—with core stabilization available, an inner ear that works, with peripheral vision available, for example. With all this, we will have the orientation to support our potential of action, providing some of the backdrop for effective action. These functions can be loosely grouped into body schema—not a simple place in the brain but a complex function. Or we can simplify and call this an "axis"—an imaginary support (Montreux workshop, 2009).

In this model, the body image comes in as a different though related function: the awareness of what happened in the past, the history, my security, the sense of wholeness that is like an envelope, a skin, around me. Hubert would say: "We need to give this sense of the envelope through our touch. Through the way we touch, we respect the fact of the integrity of the person's sense of territory. We accept that the territory comes toward us and that reopens the possibility of a secure envelope."

This is the direction I take as a practitioner today in response to Benjamin's words.

"Feel what you are touching right now," I suggest. "The way the table feels under your back, the pillow meeting your head. Can you feel the touch of the blanket on your skin?" I ask. I pause to give him a chance to notice.

I point out:

> The skin is the biggest organ; it's the real boundary of inside and outside. A sense of our literal skin can be really helpful in feeling safer, less likely to be invaded. When you don't have enough sense of skin, the world can seem overwhelming. Long ago, I had dreams of being a baby with no skin—of being unable to screen anything out. The imagery of a whole skin and the sensory response it evokes have been very helpful for me.

I pause again.

> When there isn't enough of that sense of the skin as a boundary, in order to feel safe, you have to make a second skin out of tensing your muscles. Instead, if you notice the points of contact, the sensations of meeting at the skin with the table under you, with the blanket that's covering you—if you pay attention to that information, you may not need so much tension.

Hubert often referred to Didier Anzieu's 1995 book, *Le Moi Peau*, which explores this phenomenon in depth.

I continued:

> Your system is always selecting information from the environment, choosing what to pay attention to. Of course, if you don't feel a real boundary, the real skin membrane that surrounds you, you have to create one. If you have that membrane, then the world actually can help you define yourself. We know ourselves in that meeting, at the surface or interface.

Dropping into this experience, Benjamin quietly said, "My mind is blown. I'm going to have to take this home with me." Recognizing that choice was involved, that he could direct his attention, finding this in the very moment, was deeply moving.

To end the session, I asked him to walk around the room, experiencing his new sense of being there, the differences in his sense of self and sense of relationship from the beginning of the session. When a person stands up from the table and begins to walk around the room, they get a chance to bring their experience into action, oriented in the space. We don't want to leave them in the interoceptive stream without adding this important step of integration. They have to integrate their experience by moving in the world.

Benjamin reported that he felt different, centered and free, that his shoulders didn't hurt. He said he could hear the sounds in the room and welcome them in. He observed that when he started to feel overwhelmed with that kind of sensory information, he could come into the place of contact of his feet with the ground, or he could feel the air moving with his skin, as if he were walking through fluid.

Then I asked him if he could find his old way again. Why would I want him to revisit his old posture? Wouldn't that risk messing up the new one? That is often what people worry about, and I don't insist if they don't feel comfortable. As we saw in the session with Carol in Chapter Six, posture and attitude go together. They are inadvertently practiced on a regular basis. But if we take the time to become familiar with how we do what we are doing, we increase our options. The moment between standing up from the table and going out into the world is a great opportunity to bring our strategies into consciousness. It allows a person to actually feel how they meet the world, what they choose to pay attention to, how they shape their attitude, and the different perceptual choices available to them.

The presence of another person allows simple witnessing or may offer another integration opportunity: bringing the movement into relationship with another person. Moving with another person is an additional step to integration—bringing these options into life. I asked Benjamin to use his old way while he looked at me. He pulled himself into his "held" posture, his usual attitude, and looked at me with great expectancy. To me, it conveyed "trying to please"—how he felt around his boss, he had mentioned during our session. But when he reshaped himself, by choosing to rest into the floor and rest into his skin, his demeanor became inviting and receptive. It was a significant shift, to an attitude of welcoming. Comfortable in his own skin.

EMBODYING SKIN

TRY THIS   ✓

There are many ways we can approach activating skin sensation in an embodiment practice. Here are a few examples.

With a partner: Starting with your arm in front of you, your partner touches or gently pinches some skin at your sternum, while you open your arm to the side, allowing the feeling of expansion in the whole sheet of tissue (from sternum to wrist or fingers). Try with each side.

Then your partner gently pinches some skin at your mid-back while you bring your arm back to the starting position. Try this movement of skin on one side at a time—noticing the feeling of the front and back skin on each side.

Then try with both sides together in the simple movement of opening your arms to the sides and bringing them back to the front.

You can also use your imagination. As your arms move, feel the air on your skin; allow your focus to go from the inside of the forearm (as you open out) to the back of the forearm (as you return)—then switch your focus so you feel the back of your forearm as you open your arms, as if meeting the air.

Or try feeling as if you are moving through a substance, water, or a thicker, more viscous substance that surrounds you on all sides.

Or, in Cat-Cow, for example, you can use your imagination to activate the skin of the back surface and the front surface as you move; or have your partner gently touch the skin at the apex of the thoracic curve or take a little skin gently between thumb and forefinger at the apex of your lumbar curve and your cervical curve during the movement.

LAYERS OF IMAGE: BODY IMAGES IN DEVELOPMENT AND CULTURE

The term "body image" covers over layers of complexity that are rarely made explicit. For Head and Holmes, body image was about the conscious representation of body in contrast to the body schema, the unconscious part. But for those of us working with body/mind, movement, and psyche, body image is by no means entirely conscious. In a 2009 workshop in Montreux, Switzerland, Hubert described three layers of body image we experience: our earliest sense of ownership through interoception; the body image we develop in relation to others; and the metaphors and symbolic language that shape our experience (Anzieu, 1995; Dolto, 2014;

Nasio, 2007). Distinguishing layers of body image allows us to refine our approach in practice with ourselves and our clients.

First body image: Interoceptive pathways

One body image, the earliest from a developmental point of view, arises from interoceptive messages, sensory signals from the viscera that refer to basic needs: feeling hungry or thirsty, cramping, et cetera. Hubert described these interoceptive messages as the basis of a body envelope, a body that needs protection. "With the body schema alone," he reminded us, "there was no territory; but now a territory appears, an envelope appears: the first body image, in the sense of the security of myself as volume" (Cadiz workshop, 2013). The newborn begins to develop a body image, a sense of territory to protect. This is the most primal body image we experience, the sense of body as ownership. It's literal: our sense of weight, the feeling of being a volume, whole and intact. When things go well during this formative phase, the first body image is the basis of a sense of security. It's a shell in the positive sense—a semi-permeable boundary with no holes.

But if there has been some trouble in this early developmental phase, there are many ways to work with re-establishing a sense of wholeness or volume. For instance, Hubert told of anorexic patients who greatly benefited from wearing a light-weight scuba suit: the slight tension/touch all over may feed the needed sense of security from the skin (Grunwald & Weiss, 2005). He also suggested that when rehabilitation is done in water, the contact of the water with the whole body may contribute to regaining a sense of wholeness after an injury or surgical procedure. Normally, the benefit is attributed to the water's resistance, which would lead to a mechanical increase in strength. Hubert suggested a less obvious healing: that the body image was nurtured through the touch of the water on the whole surface of the skin.

When Sherrington coined the term "interoception" in 1906, he wanted to contrast sensory information coming from inside the body (sensations from the viscera) and sensations coming through the skin from outside— temperature, pain—which he called exteroception. More recently, Bud Craig furthered our understanding through his pioneering research on interoceptive pathways (Craig, 2015). Craig points to extensive research showing that the skin is filled with small-diameter axons (look back at the chart in Chapter Ten) that communicate the state of the tissue itself. Using microelectrodes, Craig followed a neuron from the spinal cord to the brain, tracking a pathway that exists only in primates. With a clear basis in functional anatomy, interoception's importance is beginning to be recognized in diverse fields, from neuroscience to psychology to sports and education.

The interoceptive stream of information signals areas in our brains, resulting in a general sense of feeling on the simple level mentioned earlier—pleasant or unpleasant, arousing or calming. It represents the tissues of our body, including bone, skin, muscle, and viscera.[1] It is not the same pathway as the one that feeds the somatosensory cortex. It's different from touch and balance and proprioception. The interoceptive pathway conveys to the brain the feelings (sensations) that we have emotions *about*, such as pain. Craig adopted Sherrington's term interoception and added skin sensation as well as input from the viscera to its definition. These days, scientists and therapists also include neurotransmitters and the input of cranial nerves to the interoceptive streams of information. Many streams of internal information feed our sense of body, of what constitutes "me."

In her book *How Emotions Are Made*, Lisa Feldman Barrett offers this definition: "Interoception is your brain's representation of all sensations from your internal organs and tissues, the hormones in your blood, and your immune system" (Barrett, 2018, p.56). Barrett furthered Craig's work, connecting interoceptive information with what we call emotion.

The work of these researchers provides supporting evidence for a direct body/mind connection, the sensory information that creates a sense of self. Ian was able to use interoceptive information to locate himself to some extent.[2] But recall Ian's experience in the MRI machine, the anxiety that arose when he couldn't tell where he was. His account suggests that interoception is not enough to provide a sense of security. Perception of the environment, where I am, or orientation—the foundation of action—must be included.

Second body image: Mirror stage

The second layer of body image that Hubert described to us is related to the French psychoanalyst Jacques Lacan's mirror stage (Lacan, 1966). Initially considered a phase we experience from six to 18 months of age, Lacan's concept evolved to name an important aspect of our sense of self. To see ourselves as a whole, we have to imagine someone else's point of view: I see another's back, so I reason that I must have one, too. To imagine my own back, my wholeness, I have to take the point of view of another person, looking at me. In this way, our "self" image is the image of an Other. When Benjamin looks at me expectantly, he is imagining himself seen in my eyes. He is no longer based in his own sensations alone, but rather includes the imaginary—how he imagines my seeing him.

The mirror of the Other

In the mid-1990s, when the first research on mirror neurons was published, Hubert mentioned how important it would turn out to be. "Ramachandran says it's the most important research to come out this year," he told us.[3] In the first experiments involving monkeys, researchers found that the activity of certain neurons changed not only when the monkeys ate a banana themselves but also when they watched a researcher eat a banana. Further research confirmed that observing an action in another activated the same motor representation in the observer (Gallese *et al.*, 1996). At the time, this was a dramatic finding, turning much of accepted neuroscience on its head.

A 2009 study looked at another dimension: that of movement restriction. Researchers in Germany showed that just seeing a picture of another person's hand on a table with two fingers restrained by small metal clamps slowed the observer's response time when they were instructed to move those same fingers (Liepelt *et al.*, 2009).

Hubert elaborated on this research: "I am alone, the capacity of my arms to move, the speed and the efficiency is measured." He explained that if he then sat in front of a handcuffed workshop attendee:

> My own capacity to move will also be diminished! If I do the very same measurements, the results will be lower. The movement of my arms is not just from me, but also from the social group that is around me. My capacity for movement is shaped and affected by the place I live, the people around me. This is the second definition of body image, it's the imaginary, the relationship with our surroundings, with the Other. (Montreux workshop, 2009)

The body seems to be most personal, most essentially "me." Hubert reminded us that the second layer of body image includes the Other. The research on how witnessing another person's constraints could change my body's experience suggests a reimagining—our body experience as porous rather than impermeable, impacted by the Other directly and physically, not just in the emotional sphere.

These first two layers of body image are never identical. One is a sense of our body from interoception, or from our own sensations or through touch. The second is an image of an Other that comes in from outside. My back is a reflection of yours that I see. You are the mirror. Inside and outside begin to break down as clear categories. Right from the beginning, before self-consciousness begins, the body image is imaginary, an interpretation, a construction. It's not a given but rather an ongoing creation, and that means it can be deconstructed and can change.

Third body image: The body of metaphor

The third layer of body image that Hubert introduced is the symbolic body, which is linked to language. He gave an example of the impact of body metaphors on our sense of self. In French, the colloquial term for cleft lip is *bec de lièvre*: a hare with a beak, a combination of two creatures, unnatural. But in Chinese culture, the colloquial term is "lotus flower": an appealing image from nature. The lotus flower represents beauty and purity. The different symbolic association leads to a different imagining, a different feeling. Symbolic language is also a dimension of body image. If we listen, the language a person uses to refer to their own body gives us clues to their symbolic process, how they imagine "body."

Embodying images

In practice, in a session, the three layers of body image Hubert described happen together. Inside/outside, self/other, how we translate our experiences into words, and how we take in the world, all shape us. They are all part of what we see and experience, our embodiment.

The session with Benjamin shows another aspect of perceptual strategy in addition to the examples in previous chapters with Fred and Gene, Ian and Sy. Throughout the day, we manage instability to stay upright, and we organize streams of information from various sources, internal and external. Mostly below the level of consciousness, moment to moment, we choose what to pay attention to and coordinate these various levels of perception as we go about our days. We can ask these questions:

- Do I have enough support or backing to allow contact?
- Do I have plasticity to find the right tool for the job, so to speak, or to shapeshift to fit the current situation?

Seeing from this perspective is the somatic basis for what tends to be named "psychological." The questions above can be read both literally and metaphorically.

> **TRY THIS** ✓
>
> Explore your associations with support or backing, journaling or as a meditation. Is your inclination more metaphorical or more literal? If you haven't already, explore these questions literally: where is your support coming from at this moment? Since you are not falling over, you are using some means of support.
>
> Can you follow your embodied experience as you detect how you are getting support right now?
>
> Can you detect any unnecessary effort you may be using? What happens if you let that go?
>
> Does the answer to the question "What is supporting me?" change?

The layers of body image described earlier are themselves interpretation. The implication is that *reinterpretation* is possible. In recognizing the meanings we are giving, we can try other options: for example, instead of physically bracing in anticipation of another's negative response— "Uh-oh, this is going to be hard!"—we can rest into the ground, seeking a sense of rooting, or sense the space around us. This prepares us for a different action and a different outcome. We can experiment with choosing different perceptual pathways to positively impact our responses in different contexts. In any given moment, we have a range of options, for example:

- We could drop into interoceptive pathways to find out how we are feeling.
- In meeting the eyes of the Other, we could come back to our own sensations or location, where we meet the world.
- We could practice slowing down to allow ourselves to notice the quality of this meeting.
- Or we could let go of trying any strategy in order to discover what is available, here and now.

These approaches may seem familiar to those who meditate. Yet, by understanding the physical mechanisms involved, we can keep our meditation from drifting away from the physicality of the present moment.

The distinction between interoception and action space is also important. The inside feelings—the interoceptive track—provide important information for knowing how we feel emotionally: whether we are feeling anxious or excited or scared, interpretations of how activated our nervous system is. But walking in the world is the domain of body schema, of orienting, of action. It gives us a different kind of security. The more we understand the elements of perception and orientation, as well as the very physical, basic level of emotion—the way we construct and interpret to make sense of the world—the more creativity we can bring to creating a sense of ease in spite of changing circumstances.

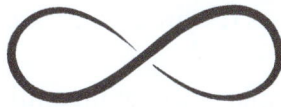

A MOVEMENT MYSTERY

American philosopher Shaun Gallagher returns to the case of Ian Waterman in his book *How the Body Shapes the Mind* (2005). We have followed Ian's process of learning to use vision and elaborate routines to accomplish the seemingly simple movements that most of us would take for granted such as picking up a cup. Over time, Ian also learned and rehearsed how to control his gestures when telling a story. As long as he could see his hands, he could carefully orchestrate their movements to match what he was saying.

At a later point, Gallagher conducted an experiment in which Ian sat in a chair with his hands hidden by a screen. Without vision, normally Ian would not be able to move. Gallagher got him to tell a story and watched as Ian's hands and arms moved automatically, for the most part as yours or mine would. It was quite a surprise to discover that when in animated conversation, Ian's hands moved on their own as he was expressing himself. Ian was unaware of what his hands were doing. Given his lack of sensory feedback, when the screen hides Ian's hands, it shouldn't be possible for his movements to happen in an organized way. But that's what Gallagher saw.

Gallagher could see a clear difference in the coordination of the movements with and without the screen. When Ian could see his hands, his movements were deliberate. The pace of his speech slowed to match the movements, which were themselves slower. There was more jerkiness and less flow in their organization. When Ian couldn't see his hands, the movements were natural and flowing—their kinetic melody intact.

What's our takeaway from this unexpected observation? Like the blind children who spoke with their hands described in Chapter Nine, Gallagher's experiment suggests that expression may be a special kind of motor act. There is more to movement than practical actions in the world, and there is a lot left to discover.

Is there an expressive motor system that has some independence from our deliberate intentions? Time will tell. Understanding the complex processes involved in movement is a work in progress, not a done deal. Regardless of the outcome, as research progresses, it provides us with new ways of imagining ourselves.

Part IV continues the exploration of imagining in relation to embodiment, how we work with perception and imagination in practice, and how we imagine the action space which includes our inherent relationship with our surroundings.

IMAGINING

CHAPTER FOURTEEN

Embodiment Practices

PERCEPTION AND IMAGINATION

In the 19th century, the German physician and physicist Hermann von Helmholtz (1821–1894) explored how the brain interprets sensory information. At that time, he made a distinction between bottom-up processes—ones that are hardwired—and top-down processes—what we add through memory and experience. While the brain is more complex than the opposition of bottom-up and top-down implies, researchers in modern times continue to refine and expand this model to capture how perception works.

We use both of these systems to solve the problem of how to interpret the world. Bottom-up, innate rules guide us to extract useful information from images, such as "contours, intersections and the crossing of lines and junctions" (Kandel, 2016, p.22). But top-down processes play a bigger role in our interpretation of visual and other sensory information than most of us realize. When confronted with ambiguous information, our nervous system fills in based on previous experience and associations.

In his 2016 book *Reductionism in Art and Brain Science*, the neuroscientist Eric Kandel borrows the term "the beholder's share" to describe what the viewer brings to the perception of a work of art and to everyday experience (Kandel, 2016, p.18). Originating from the ideas of art historian Alois Riegl and philosopher Ernst Gombrich at the turn of the 20th century, the beholder's share emphasizes that perception is not a passive process but an interactive one.

Previous experience, anticipation, and prediction shape every perception. For example, we naturally assume that light usually comes from above, because that is what we have experienced most of our lives (the sun or ceiling lights). Visual illusions take advantage of this expectation to fool us—and reveal our assumptions. In the "bumps and hollows illusion" (CuriosityShow, n.d.), for example, when light hits a rounded object from above, the top part of the object looks brighter and the bottom part is in shadow. When you see that shading pattern—lighter on top, darker on the bottom—your brain interprets the shape as being lit from above, and that makes it look like it is bulging out.

If you flip the same circle upside down, now with the darker part on top and lighter part on the bottom, it will look like a hollow. Because if the "light" is still imagined to come from above, the part in shadow would be on top, making the shape seem as though it's curving away from you. This classic visual illusion shows how strongly our perception depends on the expectation that light comes from above.

Culturally, we take perception and perceptual processes for granted. We don't realize that we *learned* to perceive. Although we don't expect children to automatically know how to read, or to play the piano or tennis, for example, we assume that perception is a given. This attitude is so far from the way it actually works! In reality, perception is an act of creation in which the incomplete information from the world is filled in by each one of us in our own way. Memory and imagination are inherently part of perception.

Perception is constructed of many elements: combining sensory information from inside and outside, filtered by our selection and interpretation of the information. It is based on associations that connect many brain regions. Visual areas of the brain recruit other areas that process touch and emotion[1] (Kandel, 2016; Salomon *et al.*, 2016). Even color itself is evocative. The inferior temporal cortex contains regions which specialize in processing information about color, and also connect with the hippocampus and amygdala which bring in emotion. Whether I am looking at the room I am in or an abstract painting, I am adding in an interpretation that combines multisensory experience as well as emotional associations.

The power of abstract painting lies in the beholder's share. Kandel suggests that the lack of representation leaves more room for our creativity as our top-down processes respond to shape, line, and color. The simplicity allows the experience to reflect the viewer's associations. Abstract artists such as Mark Rothko eventually abandoned all images for color fields alone to great effect. The canvases on the walls of the Rothko Chapel in Houston are painted shades of brown, black, and plum. No fixed light illuminates the paintings. Instead, a large skylight with its changing light stream allows the paintings to remain responsive to the moment of the viewer's perception. Imagination and perception meet; an emotion arises. For one person, it may be a sense of timeless serenity. For another, there is a sense of movement—that could be in the painting or in the person viewing. From a neuroscientific perspective, perception, emotion, and imagination are deeply intertwined, relying on overlapping neural networks and cognitive processes (Kandel, 2016).

Could the delight of embodiment practices share some of what Kandel describes in the experience of abstract art—a multisensory experience that allows imagination to bring us something new?

The next few chapters explore ways of imagining ourselves in movement through embodiment, research, and a case study. Imagination enters into emotion and into our perception of our surroundings—the action space. How do imagination, emotion, and action operate in embodiment, in theory, and in practice?

TWO EXAMPLES: EFFORTLESS ACTION AND THE REALM OF VOLUMES

From 2008 through 2011, a colleague organized a series of five French-language workshops for somatic practitioners in Switzerland. With a consistent group of students over the course of three years and speaking his native language, Hubert was able to address complex topics of perception, psychology, and neuroscience with greater fluency than in the previous workshops I had attended.

The first workshop in the series took place in December 2008, in the mountain town of Chandolin: an ancient alpine village resting in a valley 6000 feet above sea level. Impacted by the altitude, I remember feeling short of breath trudging uphill through the snow to the hostel and classroom. I waited all week and finally the clouds parted to reveal the stunning view of the Alps.

From the first day of the workshop, along with relevant research on perception and biomechanics, Hubert continued to present us with movement practices that evolved our experience of the many facets of embodiment.

To many in the bodywork community, lying on a table or on the floor and getting in touch with interoceptive information is hugely appealing. But to me, focusing on the interoceptive stream often felt overwhelming and disorienting. Because lying down and feeling stuff inside was often assumed to be a positive experience, it was hard for me to even articulate what I felt uncomfortable about. I surmise that I am not entirely alone in this.

Hubert's approach was a rare combination. He provided terms that we could use to describe our own and our clients' experiences. He took the time to explore the complex concepts in neuroscience and psychology. Then he would lead us through embodiment practices that helped make embodied sense of the theory while helping us to build a capable body, responsive and well oriented. For me, Hubert's integrative approach was a godsend. Rather than being told to just trust in experience, I was learning to find a comfortable orientation, both physically and intellectually.

"Body work," somatic work, can be movement work, a work of both sensing and imagining, exploring the capacities that lead to a change in how a person feels in the world. Perceptual processes—which include the imaginary—are a way to enter into an exploration of embodiment. Here are two examples from the Swiss workshop series. Through these embodiment practices, we were able to integrate the theory of body schema and body image.

EMBODIMENT PRACTICE 1: NON-DOING—EFFORTLESS ACTION

Effortless action: I had many times heard this esoteric paradox, a principle in Chinese philosophy and martial arts. Hubert's understanding of the science of movement provided the underpinnings to turn this appealing idea into an embodied experience.

We sat on chairs arranged in a circle. Sliding towards the front of his chair, Hubert invited us to do the same, to come to the edge of the chair and feel that we were rolling towards the very front of the pelvic bones (the ischial tuberosities, the "sitting bones"). He guided us to put our weight *in front* of the sitting bones, where the hamstrings are said to attach. Using this starting point, I felt that as I let go, my weight fell forward directly into my feet, into the ground. As the weight dropped into the floor, it was easier to feel the floor through the soles of my feet (what Hubert called "increasing the hapticity"). I also felt an effortless rebound, a response of support around my spine that still left me free to move.

Then Hubert suggested we place our hands on our thighs, fingers pointing towards each other, and asked us to feel the spine sliding between the shoulder blades, forward and back. He reminded us that in this part of the exercise the shoulders themselves don't move. He explained that this way the muscles of core stabilization around the spine would automatically engage: when I go forward, the multifidus muscle—the deeper, local spinal muscles—are activated, and when I go back, they relax—without trying![2]

Then he asked us to feel the tiny movement—only three degrees—of the sacrum between the two hip bones (the ilia). Not so easy! To help us, Hubert suggested first to rock the whole pelvis forward and back, so we could feel ourselves moving the sitting bones, the whole pelvis. Then we tried to keep the pelvis still, while the spine moved between two stable hip bones. We don't usually make these careful distinctions in our movements. Hubert called the change in what moves and what stays still "changing the fixed point." "This is your sacro-iliac joint," he told us. He cautioned, "Beware of using hip muscles: the movement we want is all in the spine."

These subtle differentiations allowed us to discover not *how to move*, but *what we could let go of*. They made us aware of tensions we had not previously perceived—what we were holding on to and what we could let go. Seeking a feeling of free movement for the sacrum requires finding how to let go of the tension around the tailbone (coccyx). If there's too much tension around the tailbone, the back of the pelvic floor will restrict the spine's movement. Along with the micro-tensions we hold in our necks (to keep our perspective, so to speak), letting go of holding in the back half of the pelvic floor makes a huge difference in our attitude, our options. The images—*because anatomy is an image!*—combined with the movements to help each one of us find the restrictions in our own bodies, restrictions we were so used to that we didn't even notice them anymore. As we let go of the habitual holding, new movement possibilities emerged.

From here, Hubert encouraged us to fold at the hip joints, again making a subtle but revealing distinction: this time, the femurs are the fixed point,[3] and the two halves of the pelvis (the ilia) move on the heads of the femurs. This movement is much easier if there is freedom in the back of the pelvic floor—another example of initiating movement by letting go. If the muscles around the tailbone are tight, it will also restrict the two hip bones' movement in relation to the femurs.

Coming back, we don't let our tailbones touch the chair. Hubert offers an image: "It's almost as if there was an internal motor for the spine, and that's what is moving."

Then, from the same starting position, sitting, spine circles: starting from a c-curve, using the image of the snake rising in response to the snake charmer's music, the cobra, to lead us up to sitting. On the way back down into the c-curve, moving slowly enough to feel the movement of one vertebra at a time. Hubert explained again that the process of imagining (or feeling for) the possibility of moving one vertebra at a time is a way to access the muscles of core stabilization. "The experience is that the movement is not my doing it, or my will," he said. "It's the feeling that something is moving. It's almost surprising to find or discover the movement instead of doing it."

All these movements take the bones as a starting point. They are an imagining of the body as bones and joints. We don't focus on performing a movement; rather, we imagine the articular relationships, the articulated body, and a sense of directions in space (up/sky, down/ground, towards and away). Evoking these images gives us a chance to find, rather than do, the movements. Like the tuna described in Chapter One, we are finding non-doing, effortless action.

Still sitting, Hubert said, "Now taking the ribcage as a fixed point, find the tiny anterior/posterior movements of the spine/sacrum, and coccyx, letting the hip bones move this time. It's not a big movement at all."

He continued:

The issue with movement is how do we get there—where do we come from? Whatever exercise we do, we want to reach the anticipatory level. Otherwise, we are really just repeating our attitudes; the pre-movement has already put its stamp.

The question Hubert began with was how to access a different pre-movement. We take a different starting point, a different strategy: letting go to move, instead of trying to make something happen. We can start with a different image, a different metaphor. For example, we imagine being on a horse and following the horse's movement. Or we can change the way the weight is resting or how we are in touch (*haptos*). Are we able to receive the touch of the floor?

Getting unstuck from our old way of doing is harder and more important than trying to figure out the right way to move; moving will always depend on the context and is better left to lower brain areas. We want to find a place to start from that allows the new to appear.

Hubert continued: "The sacred word of movement: *non-doing*." At last, the appealing idea of non-doing became a felt experience through this embodiment practice. Feeling strong did not require the feeling of effortful contraction, the exertion of willpower, or a no pain/no gain attitude. Effortless action arose through finding a different pre-movement, which starts with a perceptual selection. We wait. We use metaphors like the cobra rising. The body schema may be out of our voluntary control, but it is not out of our influence if we know what to pay attention to: weight resting into the surface of chair and floor, finding support in the meeting places with the world around us (ex-proprioception). All the theory related to the perceptual body that has been outlined in the previous chapters comes to bear in effortless action. Imagination is a part of it: in this case, the imagery involves the articular system, a sense of where our weight rests and of where we are going. We can take as a starting point that our ribcages are attracted to our friends on the other side of the room. Our friends become the supporting image for our chests, so the hips are free to move. We begin to include the other in our embodiment, free to move towards or away.

In this way, theory informed practice. We were practicing how to choose a different starting point, to find another way to initiate movement. We were developing perceptual plasticity, variability instead of one right way. Using the imagery of the bony relationships supported moving with less voluntary contraction, helping us to find the movement, not do it. Our focus was less personal, more about vectors and moving in space.[4] We were choosing the information that would best allow the body schema to be free to do its job.

EMBODIMENT PRACTICE 2: VOLUMES

The next year, the workshop for French-speaking Rolfers met again in Switzerland, this time in Montreux, on the shores of Lake Geneva, the hometown of one of our colleagues. On the first day, we were reintroduced to the non-doing embodiment just described, as in the year before. Then on the second day, Hubert led us in a variation of the previous day's embodiment. This time the focus was on the interoceptive stream that makes up the first body image from infancy, the sense of volumes, of our own territory. Hubert used a skeleton and a medium-size ball to illustrate. Placing the ball inside the pelvic bowl (the two ilia and the sacrum), he invited us to change the fixed point again.[5] This time, we were to imagine the ball as a substitute for the organs (viscera) that occupy that space inside the pelvis.

If you want to try this as you read, as in the previous embodiment, start sitting forward on the chair.

Sitting, Hubert invited us to feel that we were rolling towards the very front of the pelvic bones (the ischial tuberosities, the "sitting bones"). He guided us to put our weight *in front* of the sitting bones, where the hamstrings are said to attach.

Hubert reminded us of the movements we had done the day before. Today, we would do the same movement, but instead of focusing on the articulations (the joints, the bony relationships), we were to imagine the freedom of the visceral space.

"Imagine a ball, a ball with sphincters, and we will try to move like yesterday, forward and back around the ball, without putting any tension in the ball," Hubert explained. *"Sometimes it can feel like there are places where the little ball is too attached to the skeleton; there are suspensory ligaments that aren't free. The ball should have some independence."*

We spent some time exploring for ourselves whether we could feel the effect of this different image, an image of a volume.

It's unusual to start a movement from this point of view, imagining our internal physical space. Can I imagine/feel the whole pelvis, the bones moving around the ball without interfering with it? We are taking a different starting point so we can find a different way to move. In changing the fixed point, the image calls upon the literal flesh, the tissue, differently. The artificial distinction between the physical/real and the imaginary dissolves.

Then Hubert invited us to begin to pay attention to the sphincters in the space from pubic bone to tailbone. Although this can be an emotionally charged area, the simplicity of the anatomical terms helped us find a neutral place from which to investigate the movement possibilities of this intimate space.

Hubert spoke slowly, naming each area to allow us to notice in detail, using our attention and small movements to influence our body image. *Follow along with these directions, trying them out for yourself, starting from sitting towards the front of your chair, forward on your sitting bone:*

"Between the coccyx and the anus, does the space lengthen both on the right and the left? What impact does this area have on movement as a whole?"

"Then between the anus and the vagina, or the anus and the scrotum (during delivery of babies, it's an area that can often be impacted). Imagine the ball with the sphincters like doors; can they open and close?"

Hubert described a fluid feeling: "The sphincters can be defended sometimes, so we are seeing if we can open or close each space of the perineum. Each space has an impact on the freedom of movement of the spine (in the sagittal plane)."

Hubert went on in the geographical exploration of the floor of the pelvis from back to front: *"Between the vagina and the urethra—it really doesn't matter if you don't have a vagina, because it is imaginary,"* he said.

"We are using the imaginary to explore. Imaginary is different from image: imaginary is created anew each time."

He continued: *"Then between penis and pubis. This is a zone that has a big impact on body image, so we are going slowly, one zone at a time, exploring if we can feel/imagine each of these spaces. And then coming back to letting the skeleton roll around the ball inside the pelvis."*

Then Hubert suggested we notice the impact this exploration had on the soles of our feet. Although it may come as a surprise to link the foot and the pelvic floor, in the brain's body map, the two areas are close together. In walking, restrictions in the floor of the pelvis impact the foot. With incontinence, for example, trying to hold the sphincters will cause tension in the foot. With the tension, Hubert described it "as if the foot disappears" as a source of support when in contact with the floor.

We went on to a similar exploration, imagining another space, another ball in the abdomen. This is the space of the digestive organs, surrounded by the peritoneum, the connective tissue membrane that enfolds the digestive system, and the kidneys, which are behind, outside the peritoneal space. This abdominal ball slides on the iliacus muscles that line the two iliac bones.

Hubert asked: "Can the two balls, the volume in the pelvis and the one in the abdomen slide on each other?" And then we went on to explore whether the skeleton—the lumbar spine, in this case—could move around the ball of viscera. The spine was moving, but the feeling was different from that of yesterday's embodiment of the articular body. Today we were imagining internal space, the water balloons rolling over each other, and the spine in relation to these volumes.

"Can you move the skeleton all around the peritoneum?" Hubert asked. *"We are not thinking of musculoskeletal as the support system now, but the visceral instead. Is there space between the peritoneum and the lumbar spine? And then the diaphragm (which is above the abdominal ball)—is it free to slide on the ball of abdominal viscera? And in the back, can the kidneys slide on the psoas?"*

We followed the embodiment up to the diaphragm to feel for freedom around the bony landmarks and organs, and went on to the lungs—the inside of the ribcage—and to the brain. As with the movements we did the day before, we can't do this internal exploration with the same voluntary contractions we might normally use to move. To find these possibilities, we have to find permission to feel our borders, our territory, to feel if we could or wanted to open (or not) to the outside.

There were differences between the feeling of action of an articular body that can almost disappear in a sense of direction/vector, a sense of meeting the world (ex-proprioception), and the feeling of movement with our focus on the visceral body. We had changed the image of the body, and we had moved to a different domain. We were not in the action system anymore. We were not ready to move, but we had explored our territory, including the forbidden areas, to locate zones that are open and ones that may feel closed.

We finish by imagining how the different volumes roll on each other. We add the thigh, the calf. Although the limbs don't technically have a visceral space, Hubert asked us if we could imagine them as volumes. Perhaps not imagining the muscular quadriceps or the bony femur, but a different quality, the volume of the leg.

He said: *"And in the foot, what is the internal volume that the foot can roll around? Perhaps putting more attention on the skin of the foot than on the muscles or bones."*

Then Hubert invited us to look at the person sitting across the circle from us, to see how our movement experiment had changed the sense of relationship. As we come to look at each other, we found ourselves in a different realm from our usual action orientation. We were in a place of continuity, fluidity. That's the interoceptive domain.

Hubert continued: "So then the question becomes whether I can see the other person while having this big interoceptive flow. Does our sense of volumes bring enough security to let us take each other's gaze because it isn't a dagger?"

It's a good question. How does it feel to be in this different space, inside ourselves, and then to be in relationship with another person, even a friend? Each time, in classes or in sessions with clients, when we give ourselves space to notice how it feels to include the Other, it brings in a dimension of everyday life that is often missed. We forget that the feeling of body when we are alone is not the same as body with another person, who might be looking at us, or judging or welcoming, whatever way we imagine at that moment. This is the second layer of body image described in Chapter Thirteen.

Next, Hubert asked us to do the same movement of spine circles from the day before with a feeling of the volumes we had just explored, and oriented by the foot in touch with the floor and the inner ear working. He asked us to notice if we could respect all the volumes (pelvic, abdominal, the chest above the diaphragm, the cranium, and the limbs) or did one disappear when we added the two vectors provided by the foot/floor and the vestibular system? Does one volume get in trouble or get lost?

Watching us, Hubert noted that for some of us, compared to yesterday, the movements seemed easier, more organized than they did when we did them as a bone/muscle action.

Then Hubert invited us to come into standing. Could we do this without losing the volumes?

He added the challenge of walking towards a classmate and giving that person a little push, with no resistance from them. Could we notice whether a volume closed?

Gathering together again, we exchanged our insights from the embodiment practices.

ELEMENTS OF EMBODIMENT PRACTICE

I described these two movement experiences in detail to convey how the imaginary can be a precise tool to change body image and movement, and not just a vague fantasy. Normally, we think that there is only one body, one way of being a body, or one way of being ourselves—or at least that's what I assumed. But I could feel for myself the difference in embodying the articular body and the body of volumes.

These two movement experiences also demonstrate many dimensions of what is involved in embodiment. We can come from different starting points. In the first, we explored non-doing, moving from the joints or articulations and finding vectors in space, the body of action (body schema). Although, usually, power is experienced as muscular effort and contraction, here we reimagined agency and power as rooted in non-doing. In the second, we took the perspective of the body as volumes, an interoceptive exploration. We found that we could shapeshift, challenging our habitual approach to movement by using different images (body image). The different imagery had a dramatic impact on our movement

capacity and the feelings evoked in us as we moved in different relationships and activities.

Throughout my many years of study with Hubert, he often used the
sequence of exploring a new possibility on our own, then with another's
gaze, and finally bringing the movement into action: standing and sitting,
walking, or the dynamic activity of pushing someone. Each step increased
the complexity of the coordination—what we could include (e.g., volumes
open or closing), or how we found the way to meet the new situation.

These two dimensions of embodiment—the articular body and the
sense of volumes—are distinct, but they also work together. We can use
them both, in different proportions, depending on the context. We could
initiate differently, using images to encourage a change in pre-movement.
Sometimes, Hubert suggested we look at each other and initiate the
movement as if we were going towards or away from a friend sitting on
the other side of the circle or next to us. Or we might switch the focus to
moving from the sense of volume in the chest, or the belly or pelvis. The
movements might look similar from the outside, but the feeling and the
associations were different and often revealing. Some felt easy, familiar,
comfortable. Some were exciting, and some felt a little edgy.

I found that between my usual way of accomplishing actions with tension and the possibility of "non-doing"—finding an easy and strong action
with another, even a simple push—lay associations, such as what pushing
meant to me. Different actions had different meanings to me. Did I have
permission to push? To be seen? To look at others? The different meanings
mattered to the movement, and as I explored them, I found it easier to
expand my responses. This brought home that the body is always under
construction. Our bodies are built not in the usual bodybuilding sense
of muscular effort, but from the meanings and metaphors we inhabit, as
well as our physical experiences.

Hubert would give us a way in. Then by just paying attention, the
movement might happen, as if by itself. Non-doing. Restrictions, whether
physical or emotional, could dissolve in the movement or (at the very
least) be perceived instead of operating below the level of consciousness.
This latter manifestation—the moment of awareness of tensing up or
closing off—was in some ways the most valuable because we could catch
the habit in the act.

As well as impacting my own sense of embodiment, recognizing the
distinctions between the body as volumes and the articular body also
gave me more varied ways as a practitioner to approach each client. As a

somatic practitioner, I could offer dynamic practices like the first move-ment experience described here, which took place sitting and standing, and that included moving with or in front of another person to address a sense of agency. Or I could work with clients to help them find a safe way to experience the volumes that are the very earliest sense of self in infancy.

Hubert gave this example:

> For instance, if I have an experience in which my territory (envelope) has been invaded, it can carry with it a subtle sense of failure. Through movement, I can begin to find the sense of agency and feel the strength that comes from non-doing. Then, if I can stand in front of another per-son and speak from this strength, this agency, there is a chance to feel something new.

Our habitual approach, the embodiments we choose or the ones we exclude, might be from a physical or emotional wound. Or our habit might be learned, picked up from the society around us. Some people might be comfortable working out and exercising but never include their interoceptive space in their movement. Others may be articulate about emotional processes but find themselves resisting expressive movements. Or, as I described with Benjamin (Chapter Thirteen), finding a balance between the inside and outside dimensions might be troubling. For myself, in the embodiment of volumes just described, even when the focus was on exploring my inner space, I was upright and oriented, which helped me integrate the interoceptive stream. Although I never thought of myself as a dancer or an athlete, the subtle movements Hubert invited us to do spoke to me and felt safe to explore.

BODY IMAGES IN THE *ILIAD* AND THE *ODYSSEY*

The images Hubert offered of "articular body" and the sense of volumes or "body as envelope" are not random choices. In Berkeley, California, in 2002, Hubert began a workshop by pointing out that the *Iliad*—the ancient literary work that tells the story of the Trojan War—describes 240 murders but includes no word for "body." Instead of a body with inside and outside, the epic poem describes joints and articulations. There are two kinds of energy involved in movement: *menos*, in the limbs, and *tumos*, the energy of perception. All the descriptions of body are in terms of energy that circulates. "Movement was about relationship," Hubert pointed out. Language reflected this: instead of nouns such as "tree" or "rain," the relationship was embedded in the words—for example "tree-when-it-is-raining." He reminded us that the *Iliad* was composed in the time of oral transmission. By the time of the *Odyssey*, the idea of body had shifted to the sense of identity, the individual, that is more familiar to us today.

It is easy to make assumptions about the body, about movement, and about self. As we have encountered throughout these chapters, most of us have been taught to imagine the body as a machine, and our self as something quite distinct from that. We feel things "inside ourselves." We are sure that there is a me inside and a world outside. In every sentence we speak, our language tells us we are the actors, that we are in charge. *I* is the subject. Those are everyday assumptions.

Each one of us responds in our own way to the embodiment practices. To me, it was delightful to experience the articular body, not being in the volumes space as much. Non-doing, when the joint surfaces could come together, along with what Hubert called the haptic sense, being in touch, lets gravity provide the support and energy for movement. This approach felt like such an easy way to move and feel strong at the same time. Hearing about the perspective of the ancient Greeks, I was intrigued that there might have been a time when this conception of moving was the norm rather than seeming esoteric.

What goes into the sense of self has been an intriguing topic for me since I was a teenager. In college, I read existentialist philosophers, Nietzsche and Sartre, and wrote a thesis at Johns Hopkins Humanities Center (an interdisciplinary department) entitled "Self-Deception, Consciousness and the Unconscious." Later, I spent years going to week-long silent meditation retreats that provided opportunities to question my assumptions about mind and self. The embodiment processes Hubert presented, and the way non-doing actually felt, gave me a glimmer of what no-self[5] might be in action. It was a relief.

Hubert's brief description of the ancient Greeks' conception caught my attention, but it wasn't until years later that I asked him for his reference. He pointed me to *La logique du corps articulaire* (The logic of the articular body) by Guillemette Bolens, a professor of comparative literature at the University of Geneva. Bolens' book is a close reading of Homer's *Iliad* (Bolens, 2000).

What does comparative literature have to do with biomechanics, you might be wondering? Our current idea of bodies, how they work, how we move, is so ingrained that it is not easy to imagine that people may not have always seen themselves the same way we do. Like Kuriyama's comparison of ancient Chinese and Greek body images (Chapter Four), Bolens takes us to the eighth century BCE to provide a different image of body.

She writes that the *Iliad* describes in vivid detail 188 mortal wounds to the Trojans and 52 to the Greeks: eyeballs jumping out of their sockets, lances passing through the front of the neck, under the clavicle, into the shoulder (p.19). The wounds are described exactly: "The spear hit where the thigh turns in the hip; the rim (cotyle) was crushed, and two tendons were torn" (p.16). The particular joint connections that ruptured are named. The sites that are pierced are named: where the skull meets the spine, the leg beneath the knee, or the ankle, or tendons of the feet (p.21). Fingers are the only joint left unnamed (pp.31–37), according to the six-page list she compiled of every anatomical location in the text. Through Bolens' careful and beautiful descriptions, it becomes clear that the Greeks had a complete vision of anatomical relationships.

Bolens points out how peculiar it is, considering the *Iliad*'s overall anatomical specificity, that in its 15,693 verses, there is no word for body the way we use the term today. How would Homer have said "I wash my body" or "the spear entered his body?" she asks. There is *soma* (eight times), which is often used for corpse, the part left over while the psyche heads off to Hades, the underworld. Or *demas*, which means stature, or *chros*, which refers to a wrapping. The rest of the time, the text refers to limbs or joints: the body isn't referred to as unitary, only as a plurality. The *Iliad* depicts the body as bones in relation to one another, connected with tendons, a network of relationships—what Bolens calls the articular body (2000, pp.55–59).

In another passage, the text tells us that the spear point breaks the bone of the pelvis—specifically the part in contact with the head of the femur—and that tendons are torn; and only after that are we told the skin is broken. It is not an accurate rendition of what happens in time when a projectile hits a body: first, the skin is ruptured, then the bone breaks (p.22). This close reading is what gives Bolens' book its title: the *logic* of the articular body. Bolens shows us that the ancient Greeks saw the bony relationships as most important. When a hero dies, he is disarticulated—the tendons are severed. The knees come "untied," undone in death, no matter where the spear actually entered his body (p.40).

Mobility is key to heroic action. The great champion Achilleus (Achilles) is described many times through the qualities of his rapid, prompt, and agile feet. The terms Hubert quoted, *menos* and *thumos*, are what gets moving. The warriors Ajax the Greater and the Lesser notice something happening in their feet and hands, their chests. They are moved by *menos* or *thumos*, translated at times as motivation, emotion, sensory or mental, even breath and soul. The gods could get *menos* and *thumos* moving in a person. The way the text is written, the warriors didn't move themselves; they were moved. "I" receives or responds: "The thumos is moving in my chest," not "I feel the thumos" (Bolens, 2000, p.48).

This is a different body image from the one we are accustomed to, but I felt I had experienced this ancient image through the embodiment practice with Hubert. Something got moving. An intention was set, a direction was taken, and then, thanks to evolution and gravity, there was movement. The articular body is an effective mover.

From the start of her book, Bolens contrasts the articular body described in the *Iliad* with the volumes/body as envelope that appeared in later texts, such as the *Odyssey*. This more familiar body image, with an inside and an outside, is a later development. An envelope of skin defines us in so many ways today! She sees the shift in the transition from oral tradition to written (Bolens, 2001). In the oral tradition, the story was sung, told, acted out, enacted. Movement was essential to what was communicated; each rendition was unique. By the time the *Odyssey* was written down, a generation or two or perhaps even a hundred years later, a shift had occurred. The plot of the *Odyssey* turns on Odysseus' childhood nanny's ability to recognize him years later by the scar on his knee that remained unchanged. Odysseus is recognized not by his mobility, like Achilles in the *Iliad*, but by the permanent mark on his body envelope, on his skin (2000, p.10).

The image of the body as an envelope (*corps-enveloppe*) is about tension between the inside and the outside. For example, in medieval versions of the *Iliad*, when Achilles mortally wounds Hector, the gory details are of liver and lungs spilling onto the saddle—no mention of the joints and tendons of the *Iliad*. What does this subtle change tell us? The body envelope is a unit, singular. It can be cut. Its integrity depends on guts staying inside where they belong. The envelope protects us from outside assaults.

Over several centuries, the articular body of action was replaced by the body as a container. By the time of Plato (428–347 BCE), the bones' primary function was understood to be protection of the spinal cord and the brain, which were considered the organs connecting the soul with the body. There was already a hierarchy of soul (psyche) over body (soma) (pp.10–15, pp.57–58) that we are familiar with today.

When Hubert chose to give us embodiment practices that let us feel the articular body in contrast with the body envelope—the experience of volumes—he was tapping a rich source of imagery rooted in the European imagination of the body.[7] We felt for ourselves different possibilities, different behaviors, and different attitudes with each image. While we might be more in touch with our emotional pulse with the volumes, action might be easier with more focus on the articular body. There was value in exploring both options. The only idea we had to give up is that there is only one real body.

CHAPTER FIFTEEN

Action Space

OPEN THE SPACE

In Chandolin, on the workshop's third day, Hubert led us in another embodiment process. From sitting, we reached for the floor by sliding one hand down between our knees, down the inside of our leg as our gaze followed the trajectory of the opposite hand going up towards the ceiling. The end of this movement could look to the viewer like a spinal twist, but the process is much more subtle. When I tried it, it felt completely different to me to reach on the right side than on the left. Turning to the right was easy; turning toward the left, I seemed to get stuck. When I turned to the right, there was a flowing movement; no thinking, it just happened. On the left side, it was as if I met an obstacle. I didn't turn as far, and I felt stiffer.

Hubert said, "Look at Aline." I showed my movement. Our classes are very safe; there is no threat or shame in being seen. The other students and I look forward to getting clear feedback about our movement. We trust Hubert.

His instruction to me was to "open the space on the left before moving." He added: "The dancer Mary Wigman said: 'I never dance without my invisible partner.' You have to invent the space, the invisible partner, to find that part of the movement" (Bernard, 2001; Wigman, 1986, p.22).

If I stopped to think about it, I might wonder how I know what this means. When I do this movement, opening the space is something I'm imagining, but it feels very physical. In the workshop, Hubert invited us to use our senses, our hearing and even our sense of smell, to invent the space. Opening the space changes the action. The cue worked: with the next attempt, turning to the left was easy for me.

Sometimes what needs to change is how we are constructing the space.

When Hubert invited me to open the space before moving, it reminded me of a client in my own practice. Deirdre, a red-headed woman, was solidly built. She reported doing a lot of exercise. When she walked, her movements seemed to take her more side to side than forward. When I described this impression to Deirdre, she said she could almost imagine there was a wall in front of her. Instead of trying to change her movement by working the tissue directly, manually lengthening the back muscles, for instance, I suggested she imagine taking the wall away or opening a door through it. With this suggestion, her movement changed. The contralateral movement of walking—the spiraling rotation of the spinal engine—emerged (Gracovetsky, 1988). All she had to do to bring about a biomechanically more effective movement was to change how she imagined the space she was moving in. How we imagine the space we move in affects how we move.

But sometimes what is missing is the invisible partner: the Other who invites us, giving us a sense of being able to reach into our surroundings. Hubert often invokes the Other, or the second layer of body image described in Chapter Thirteen. To feel the chair that I am sitting on is to meet an Other; to feel the air or temperature on my skin is also a meeting with the Other. If we slow down enough to notice, Hubert suggests, almost any perception (interoception aside), even the sensations through the skin itself, is of the world. The world coming to us inevitably includes Other. As he often says, "Half the work is the body; the other half is about how we construct the space."

Hubert went on:

> You can't change posture if you don't change how you represent the space. It is important to emphasize this. Because in practice I find it is 95 percent of the work. It's clear that when we work with someone, we can do great work structurally with the tissue, but if we don't change the way they represent the space, and the way they represent their own posture, the problems will inevitably come back.

Deirdre and I experienced a change in our movements and the way we felt by reimagining the surrounding space, not starting from the space inside of us, nor our position, nor our muscular sense. As Hubert elaborated, there is not an inside and an outside, body and space. From a phenomenological perspective, right from the very beginning, space is a construction, a way of imagining for each person. We can't separate the body from the dynamic that constructs the space (Kuypers, 2006). To experience our body in movement this way—not as stuck inside the skin, but in relationship to our surroundings and how we imagine them—is unexplored territory for most of us. This chapter will unpack this novel idea.

AGENCY AND OWNERSHIP

The next year in the workshop in Montreux, Hubert took up the concepts of body image and body schema again to help us deepen our understanding of their implications.

In Part III, we explored the concepts of body schema and image as a way to answer the question of what body awareness is. The moving body, the process through which planning and organizing movement occurs that we designated as "body schema," is not identical to our image or idea. The moving system living in the gravitational field has constraints that may not fit the body image reflected in our personal and cultural milieu. Through our aches and pains, we discover precisely how we are living off our center. Looking in the mirror—literally or metaphorically—can't always provide a way through our troubles.

Through the embodiments that we practiced in Chapter Fourteen, we learned to shift our images. We experienced the articular body in the first practice, finding effortless action by directing our attention to weight and space (body schema). In the second practice, we explored the sense of our volumes, accessing the first layer of body image described in Chapter Thirteen. We took two different starting points, though the movements themselves—sitting in a chair, allowing the spine to flex and extend—were not that different. Each metaphor we adopt in reimagining the body lets us perceive ourselves in a different light. Like a kaleidoscope, for a moment the image arranges itself in a pattern and then, with another twist, a new pattern emerges.

The intricacies of our movement capacity are an evolving story, still in process today. During the 1990s and 2000s, Hubert sought research to make sense of his experiences working with his own embodiment and his patients' problems. At the same time, neuroscience was also developing rapidly. Hubert's genius has been to extract what is important in the new information coming from neuroscience and apply it to our movement work. Hubert's presentation of theoretical work was always drawn from practice, not concepts in the abstract. In the workshop in Montreux in

2009, Hubert presented another lens that applied in our own personal and professional practices.

That day Hubert wrote out two parallel lists on the newsprint easel: Body as Agency where body schema would usually go, and Body as Ownership on the other side where body image would be.

Body as Agency[1]	Body as Ownership
Proprioception	Interoception
Kinesthesia	Body Envelope/Flesh/Territoriality
Musculoskeletal	Viscera/Cavity
Orientation	Boundaries/Skin
Action	Security of Volume
Peripersonal Space	
Core Stabilization	

There were familiar terms on both lists along with a couple of new ones, but we had never seen them grouped under the headings Agency and Ownership. Under *Body as Ownership* in this outline were the terms we explored in depth in Chapter Thirteen (First body image: Interoceptive pathways). Hubert went on to elaborate on *Body as Agency*: "The body schema is the domain of peripersonal space, of action, of core stabilization, and orientation." Peripersonal or near space is defined as the space around us that we can reach. In the somatic field, it is also called the kinesphere (Laban, 1966).[2]

> All these aspects make up a whole system which we can call the body schema. It is the universe of proprioception: the sense of one's movements in the space—not of the body, but of the movements, kinesthesia. Perhaps the most essential discovery of recent years from a philosophical point of view, is the notion that the body schema is not identical with "the body" in the flesh. The body schema has to do with the musculoskeletal system, and it doesn't have a boundary. The body schema doesn't stop at the skin: The body schema is not the body in itself, but the body and the space that surrounds us. We integrate the peripersonal space inside of us.

Wow! What does it mean to see the body this way? What does it mean to say the body schema isn't the body in the flesh? The body schema doesn't have one fixed boundary? Through the workshop's embodiment practices previously described, effortless action became a felt experience, but this conceptualization went even further. Practitioners in many fields, from meditators to dancers and movement teachers, intuit that a sense of boundary is not unchanging, but instead is wrapped up with context and perception. Now neuroscientists' research began to provide a scientific basis for these pervasive experiences.

When I stand next to a chair that I am going to sit or stand on, the chair can be integrated into my body schema. This phenomenon is also what allows the body to accept a prosthesis. Action-based, the body schema morphs depending on what we are doing, independently of whether the device is technically "my body."

Hubert went on:

> The word "body" is truly misleading. Today, more and more scientific discoveries are going in this direction: we occupy the space around us; we can integrate the objects or not. We have to imagine the boundary of our bodies as being mobile, changing; I can be tightly squeezed, or I can occupy more space. For example, for the operator of a giant crane, his/her body schema will go the whole length of the crane—60 meters—hopefully![3]

That we can and do integrate objects into our dynamic motion really shouldn't surprise us: writing with a pen, riding a bicycle, and the way we experience the car as we are driving are familiar examples from daily life. An experienced driver has a feel for the edges of the car in relation to the curb as they are parallel parking. They may flinch when a car comes too close, as if it were their own body that was at risk of being side-swiped and not just the car's bumper. The research shows that we can integrate the boundaries of the car or other tools into the various brain areas that participate in creating the body schema (Maravita & Iriki, 2004; Spiers & Maguire, 2007). Different aspects combine and recombine depending on the specific context. Body schema is a dynamic process, not a simple, fixed, location.

Other fascinating research experiments illustrate the body schema's plasticity. In one example, researchers put the subjects in front of a screen on which a dot would appear. The subjects were instructed to touch the dot with their index finger. The precision and speed of their touch were measured. Then the subjects did the same thing with a stick of wood. When using the stick, some subjects lost their precision and others didn't at all. Using fMRI technology, the researchers were able to see whether the stick of wood was integrated into the body schema. The subjects who did not show any integration lost most of the skill they had demonstrated without the stick (Holmes & Spence, 2004).

In another study, researchers taught macaque monkeys to use a mechanical arm that was not attached to them. Tiny sensors were placed in the brain areas responsible for movement. A computer interface interpreted the signals from the electrodes implanted in each monkey's motor cortex and figured out, for example, that a certain pattern might mean "move right" or "grasp." The monkeys had to practice mastering the capacity to control the robotic arm. At first, they might make simple movements while being rewarded, such as moving their arms toward a target. With feedback (e.g., seeing the arm reach for an object and receiving a reward), the monkeys started to understand the connection between their thoughts and the arm's movements. With continued practice and adjustments, the computer program refined its ability to decode signals more accurately, and the monkeys gained better control over the robotic arm. Over time, the monkeys were able to perform increasingly complex tasks, such as grabbing a banana and bringing it to their mouths, just by thinking about it. (To watch this in action, see indoContent, 2008.) One surprising effect: once the monkeys learned to use the robotic arm, it was so easy that they stopped using their actual limb (Blakeslee & Blakeslee, 2007; Science News, 2008; Velliste *et al.*, 2008). Hubert said:

> And after a while, what happens? The monkey's actual arm degenerates, disappears. It is the opposite of the stick. Parts of the body can disappear as far as the body schema is concerned. The mechanical arm doesn't cost anything from the point of view of effort, so the monkeys can use it to get the banana, bring it to their mouths, and they stop using their own real arms—which is to say that the body schema doesn't know the body as flesh. It can add or subtract.

As we have seen, the concept we call body schema is useful but leads to some false assumptions. Body schema refers to an interconnected network of brain areas as well as feedback from the visual system and the sensory information conveyed through our skin, joints, and muscles. The monkey experiments also show that the body schema doesn't stop at our skin's boundary, but can incorporate objects—tools, cars, and also robotic arms. The body schema includes the space around us in which we take action to reach for something or to avoid something coming towards us. As far as your movement system is concerned, "you" can include a lot more than what you think of as your body. To capture some of these dimensions, Vittorio Gallese, one of the researchers who discovered mirror neurons, has suggested we replace the words "body schema" with "'source' or 'power' for action" (Gallese & Sinigaglia, 2010, p.746).

The word "body" gives the impression of something solid, fixed, and limited. Yet, in reality, the body's boundaries are mobile—not limited to the flesh we see. Hubert used the French *espace d'action*, or "action space." This was another paradigm shift for me: to no longer imagine the body as only the literal body we see—and, instead, to imagine including the surrounding space and a boundary that was always changing.

Ownership and agency were an evolution in the division of embodiment into body schema and body image. For a practitioner, this perspective is important: for example, how does this mobile boundary apply in hands-on practice? When we do hands-on work with our clients, are we integrating them into our body schema? Hubert suggested that it was possible to let our boundary go beyond our hands. Our own sense of orientation in gravity became even more important in order to avoid intruding or merging with our clients.

Outlining two realms, one of agency and one of ownership, helps inform somatic practice in another way. Over the past decades, many different approaches to healing have begun to be included in the field of somatic practice. Techniques grounded in osteopathic tradition (e.g., cranio-sacral and visceral manipulation; biodynamics and breathwork) are included as well as movement, yoga, tai chi, and meditation. As a practitioner, the concepts of ownership and agency help orient us to our client's experience. How do we know what is needed? The membranous, fluid quality in cranial and visceral work, for instance, may help to restore a person's sense of wholeness, their sense of volume and envelope, the first layer of body image. Sometimes this is what is needed. At other times, though, and perhaps within the same session, we need to address a person's sense of agency—to empower them in action. In Benjamin's session, we looked at *backing*, creating a sense of support. While initially I directed his attention to his skin boundary when he was lying down, in contact with the table, to finish the session we addressed agency through walking and connecting with each other. It's important to remember to help guide people back into action, into their orientation and agency, to go out in the world.

With the abundance of techniques available in the somatic world, it's helpful to have ways of discerning among them. In a session of cranio-sacral technique, for example, the world that is invoked is one of membranes, of fluidity, of continuity, of boundaries. A client rising from this session might not be ready to push or perform an elegant *grand jeté* in ballet.

Hubert's approach to embodiment, in which we were proprioceptively aware, always included being awake to the space. That orientation is necessary when we want to be ready for action. Hubert said:

> In a cranial session, the space matters differently because we are in a world of elements that constitute us as a volume, as a territory. But a pre-movement problem is often an action issue, about action and not about the visceral space. In addition, we are not etheric beings. We are beings who can experience fear, who can be affected, who can open or not open, who can allow the viscera to envelop the space or not. The work always goes from one to the other. You can't open the action space if there is fear dominating the interoceptive sense—the fear there will close up the space for action. And conversely, at times you have to organize the action space, the dynamic body schema, so that you can do the more psychological work. Then there is support for the body image. It will always be a back and forth between the two domains. In practice, we can work the relationship between the two.

The agency/ownership distinction gave me language to make sense of my own preferences—why I did not enjoy lying down with my eyes closed to do interoceptive practices. I preferred working with the kinesthetic approach that developed my sense of agency, of competence in the world. This shed light on my own experience with somatic practices in the past. Agency opens up the space as part of the body.

How does this work in practice? Here's an example.

CLIENT STORY: RAMONA

Finding, not doing. That was the message in the third session with Ramona.

When Ramona comes in, she still looks compressed. She works out so much and really is muscle-bound, not free. She complains of stiffness in her knee, and now the other side is hurting too, the side that wasn't operated on.

I ask her how much she works out. She says, "Oh, a lot. My personal

trainer is always watching my belly to be sure I'm using my core." Her statement makes me wonder if the way she is working out is working at cross
purposes with what we are trying to find in her Rolfing sessions—more
freedom of movement, ease, decompression.

In Hubert's perspective, "core stabilization" is not just about the belly:
it's a function that includes the whole system. All the joints need to keep
their integrity in a movement; whether the articulations need to knit
together or to let go to allow free movement depends on the circumstance.
Hubert would say that in a well-organized movement, you can't see where
the movement begins because it begins in a change of perception—that
is the beginning of core stability. You wouldn't see, for instance, a big
muscular contraction of the rectus abdominis, the "washboard" muscle.
That one just pulls your chest and pelvis together and should not be the
first to contract. Grace is when we see the movement or the expression,
not the body's shape. A dancer can have too much body, or the body can,
in a sense, disappear in a graceful movement (Chapter Eight/*Sun salute*).

Ramona seems to be using too much effort in her approach to exercise
and maybe in daily life, too. I am standing, wondering how to show appreciation for her workouts while also giving her an alternative approach: how
to help convey the idea of effortless action. "What's a way of getting this
idea across in a way that will stick?" I wonder to myself.

For some reason, call it a lucky guess or intuition, I think of *Star Wars*—a
new movie had come out recently.[4]

"Have you seen the new *Star Wars* movie yet?" I ask.

She responds, "Oh, I love *Star Wars*."

I go on. "You know how they talk about the Force?"

It occurs to me to show her "the Unbendable Arm," an exercise used in
aikido, tai chi, and other martial arts. Hubert introduced us to it during a
workshop in Philadelphia in 1993. While it might at first seem like just a cool
trick, there is substance to it. It is a change in how we perceive and include
our surroundings—a perceptual shift that changes our biomechanics.

"Here, let me show you what I'm talking about," I say. We stand facing
each other and I put my outstretched arm on her shoulder, palm up. "Try
to bend my arm," I say. "I'm going to try to stop you the usual way, with
effort." She proceeds, and we both see/feel the amount of tension and
shortening, and the many muscles that get involved in my shoulder and
neck. And while I continue to work very hard to resist, she succeeds in
bending my arm without too much trouble.

"Okay," I say. "Now I'm going to use the Force, so to speak." With my arm in the same position, palm up, resting on her shoulder, she struggles to bend it while I keep my arm extended—but this time with no visible effort. There is no question about the difference: no other muscles pop out in tension, and I don't appear to be working at all. And I'm no qi master, that's for sure.

"Wow! That is really different!" she says. "What happened? What did you do differently?"

"I'll teach you," I say. "All you have to do is imagine beams of light extending out from your fingers and beyond into the space behind me."

I explain that when we struggle, we contract both the biceps (the antagonist) and the triceps (the actual mover, the agonist that straightens the arm). This means that we are fighting ourselves, contracting muscles that work against each other and at cross purposes with our own strength (Godard *et al.*, 2001). The increased muscle tension mimics the physiology of fear. Instead of finding strength, we are almost practicing feeling afraid.

We do a version of the same process with her lying down on the Rolfing table. I stand at the end of the table as she lies on her back with one knee bent, foot on the table. She pushes the other foot against my hand. When she just pushes against me, there is a lot of extra work around her hip joint: she feels herself lift off the table, and I don't go anywhere. Much of the work she is doing just goes back into her own body, so much less force is applied in her intended direction. Then she tries it with the images that allow her to include the wall behind me, a way to let her sense of herself project out into the surrounding space. The same sense of effortless strength appears as when we were standing.

In this movement, I suggest that she feel the table under the other foot, the leg that is bent, to access her true core support. The sensation of the table meeting her foot will trigger the stabilizers in her middle so that the leg she will push with can lift up without her rectus abdominis or hip muscles triggering. The superficial muscles working too soon, before the deeper core muscles, would actually diminish the support for her action. Once support is established, the other muscles contribute extra power, but they aren't effective initiators. Like the character knot described in Chapter Seven, we will often employ the same contraction pattern in anticipation of any effort. Using a pre-movement that includes space instead of separating ourselves from it with muscle tension is another strategy to untie the knot.

As in many of the embodiments described throughout this book, "the Force" is something we *find*, not something we *do*. You can't make it happen with sheer willpower. Instead, you make contact and wait for sensations to come to you. You organize your perception of space—in this case, letting the imaginary beam of light reach through the wall. That's how you find core support.

Standing up, we try another variation. I invite Ramona to put her hand, palm down now, on my shoulder and push me. She feels how she can push by creating her familiar tension and contraction. Then she feels how she can use "the Force," this new kind of coordination that relates her to her surroundings in a different way. She feels the quiet strength of it—strength, but with ease.

I smile as I say, "Now you are a Jedi!"

The conventional viewpoint is that "body" is inside, that it needs stretching, strengthening, fixing. But in this case, and so many others, the real change comes from something different. It is a change in our relationship with our surroundings, something we do with our imagination, but that creates a change in physical reality. Is it magic, an illusion, or something else?

CLIENT STORY: JAYE—DISCOVERING THE KINESPHERE

Here's another example of using our sense of space in practice. Everyone doesn't learn the same way or need the same cue to access a new experience. It's important as a practitioner to trust what is happening. In allowing ourselves time to register the impressions of the moment, a creative response can emerge.

The first time I was invited to teach a segment of a yoga teacher training was in 2015 at Akasha Yoga Studio in Boston. At the beginning, we went around the room introducing ourselves. A well-spoken and elegant woman, Jaye, came across as strong and able to stand her ground. She described a challenging exercise that she had done with theater students in a workshop. She said that a lot of feelings were brought up for the participants and that it made the group feel unsafe. She reported that during the second attempt, they went much more slowly, and she thought they were less willing to plunge in. She raised the question: what would make it possible to open up and explore feelings and still feel safe?

Later, when Jaye and I did the Unbendable Arm exercise together, the cue that I use most commonly—to project out beyond the fingers, imagining light emitting from your fingers going out across the room in front of you—was a little more successful than when she just resisted and struggled, but not as effective as it usually is. Then it came to me to say, "Open the space behind you," and suddenly her arm was as strong as iron, and I saw the surprise in her slightly widened eyes as she felt it, too: strength without effort, an unexplored attitude. The answer to Jaye's question—how to find more safety without defensiveness—may be right here in a different use of space. Jaye found her strength by opening what Wendy Palmer, a fourth-degree black belt in aikido, calls the backfield, the part of the kinesphere behind us (Palmer, 1999, p.84). The next time she is in a difficult situation, Jaye may remember that she can change her sense of her own strength in the face of adversity by opening her backfield.

The Unbendable Arm experiment demonstrates how our body sense includes the space around us. From another perspective, it also may reveal what part of our kinesphere is missing.[5] It could be in front, but also behind, as in this example, in the backfield, or above. What's important is to understand the basic principle: that how we are imagining or constructing the space, as Hubert likes to say, is a key parameter in changing our movements.

EMBODIMENT: EMBODYING SPACE IN ALL DIRECTIONS

To embody theory, we need practices. Here is one that allows us to inhabit the idea of body-in-space. In 2002, Hubert shared this meditation with us during a workshop in Holderness, based on an experience he had long before with Tibetan Buddhist teacher Kalu Rinpoche (1905–1989), one of the first Tibetan lamas to teach in Western countries.

Sit comfortably toward the edge of the chair, feet in contact with the floor.

Imagine that in the center of your chest you have a white ball.

Take some time. It's not only a visualization; can you take the time to allow the feeling of a white ball in the center of your chest?

Not putting the white ball in a fortress, walled in; just in the center of the self, a very light, beautiful white ball, which you put somewhere in the center of the chest—and when you feel it, you hear it, you see it—with all the senses.

Then you will imagine that in front of you somewhere on the horizon there is a blue ball.

Try to be at the same level of presence with the white ball inside you and the blue ball on the horizon.

Why a blue ball? It's the quality of a blue sky.

The white ball inside is completely open to the blue ball, which means it is open to the horizon. In front of us, the visual space is completely open.

Can you notice/feel if you are more with the blue ball or with the white one?

Or can you catch a moment where you are the blue and you are the white together? You are the white ball in the center of you and you are the blue in front of you.

When it is very easy to be with both balls together (this could be many months of practice!), then imagine a yellow ball on the right side of your body, on the right horizon. And again, notice playfully: can you keep the feeling of the white ball, the blue ball, and the yellow one, all at the same time?

Does one of the three balls have a tendency to disappear in your feeling or imagining? If so, you can reinforce that one, spend a little more time there.

Step by step, you can feel there is no longer a question of inside/outside.

When you get the yellow ball, you will put a red one on the horizon behind you.

Step by step, notice if there is an interconnection between these balls.

And then we will finish the circle by putting a green ball on the left side, on the horizon.

The work of the meditation is to allow your attention not to be caught by only one ball, and instead, at the same moment, to feel/hear/smell the white ball inside you being in connection with the blue one, in connection with the yellow one, the red one, the green one.

The way we imagine our surroundings also impacts us directly through the breath. Our kinesphere and our ability to project in space shape the breath. In this meditation, the exhale will come from the white ball in the center, and the inhale from openness in all directions.

Paraphrasing Ilse Middendorf (1990), Hubert said: "Have confidence in the breath; don't do it; just have confidence that it will come on its own."

The question of inside/outside may not be the best way to frame our experience when we want to reinforce a sense of boundary. The kinesphere is the capacity of projection in space. Instead of correcting from the body, we can open the directions in space. We can reimagine our embodied experience as a projection in space, noticing which directions come easily and which need a little more attention to be accessible. In a body reading, sometimes we can see from the outside whether the body is with one ball more than the others. One direction may be strongly attracting, or one may not be very open. Remember that a change in the sense of space implies an actual change of tonus in the muscles that manage our uprightness. This is the message of the Unbendable Arm.

Hubert ended the session that day by reminding us of a story attributed to Huineng (638–713), one of the Patriarchs of the Chan school of Zen Buddhism. Two monks are watching a flag flapping in the wind. One monk says, the flag is moving; the other says, no, the wind is moving. Passing by, the Patriarch says: the mind is moving.[6]

Action Space in Research and Practice

This chapter explores working with action space—the model of embodiment that includes the perceptual patterns of orientation and action we have been exploring throughout this book—in the clinical context, first presenting Hubert's work as part of a team exploring the impact of breast cancer diagnosis on women's movement patterns and action possibilities, and second, a case study from my practice that unfolds over a series of sessions.

UNBENDABLE ARM STUDY

How do we account for the experience of the Unbendable Arm? Some people are content with calling the results "qi (or energy) flow." But for a science-minded person like me, that was not completely satisfying. Hubert's research with breast cancer patients at the Istituto Nazionale dei Tumori in Milan, Italy, went a long way towards clarifying the mystery.[1]

Initially, in the early 1990s, Hubert had been invited by the Istituto to work with the doctors' movement patterns in relation to their patients. Body reading is not usually part of medical education. I got the impression that in this hospital the doctors were thinking very differently about their patients and each other. Hubert noticed that the doctors would hold their breath when touching a patient. This unconscious action created a sense of separation, of exclusion, leaving the patient feeling more objectified. Working with this simple and profound observation made a big difference for the doctors in the department, giving them access to a change in attitude. This was just one example of subtleties that were revealed through working with the doctors' embodiment as an aspect of medical practice. Eventually, Hubert was invited to help with research using movement analysis to look into some of the problems that arose for cancer patients after breast reconstruction (see Introduction).

Over time working with the breast cancer survivors, the doctors noticed a strange phenomenon: about a year after the surgery, many of the patients were coming back with hip trouble. Because of Hubert's expertise in movement analysis, he was called in to consult about the mystery. Watching the women in motion—walking around with or without a goal, or picking up objects, and in other simple movements—he noticed that they did not move the arm on the side affected by the cancer. In particular, that arm didn't have its normal swing in walking. Hubert explored other gestures like shaking hands or pointing at specific targets (e.g., the light on the ceiling) to check the quality of movement. When asked, the women could move their arms as requested: there was no range of motion or motor deficit. There was no mechanical problem, yet something had changed in the shoulder's dynamics.

The hip trouble could be accounted for to some extent within an understanding of how arms work in walking. In walking, the swing of our arms and rotation of the trunk allow or interfere with hip motion. Over time, the change in the patients' arm movement led to a hip problem in the same or opposite hip, depending on the strategy the woman was using.

Up until that time, movement analysis of the patients had not included looking at women interacting with their surroundings, as active experiencers instead of passive subjects. Following James Gibson's ecological approach, the shift to watching the women in action made observations available that would not have shown up through the traditional assessment procedure. Hubert and the team of researchers began to track their patients' arm swing as a parameter. They discovered that in 65 percent of the post-operative women, the arm on the affected side was not engaging as much during normal activities. Then they began to check the arm swing pre-operatively—before any surgery at all—and to compare it with a sample of healthy women. Before surgery, 50 percent of the women with breast cancer showed a reduction in arm swing compared to only 10 percent of the women in the control group.

This was curious. Clearly, the change in movement was not provoked by the surgical procedure on its own. Something in the experience of finding out there was cancer of the breast impacted the range of gesture the women felt free to use. This is not an easy matter to study directly.

The clinical observation was that, post-surgery, the women were using their arms differently, which would imply a motor problem. But there was not a measurable problem when the women were asked to move their arms. Instead of being limited by a framework that divides experience into sensory and motor, Hubert and his colleagues considered the problem in Gibsonian terms of action systems and perceptual systems. From this standpoint, a missing action may imply a missing perception, a missing relationship with the environment.

In the context of a post-surgical rehabilitation group and during subsequent chemotherapy, the researchers began to investigate the women's quality of perception. They found that the women in the group were less able in both the exteroceptive and the ex-proprioceptive dimensions of perception—David Lee's elaboration on Gibson's understanding that we considered in Chapter Eleven. Hubert could see the exteroceptive trouble reflected in the weakness of the gesture of pointing—in other words, the ability to show a vector in the surrounding space. Ex-proprioception is a key aspect of the ability to organize orientation, the basis of all perception, as we saw in Ian Waterman's case. The problems in ex-proprioception showed up in the coordination of movements with the arm on the affected side, as well as in the lack of ability to anticipate an action such as catching a ball.

The researchers theorized that there might be a relationship between the emotional impact of breast cancer starting from the moment of diagnosis and the observed changes in the women's movement patterns and quality of perception. We could also describe it as a problem in haptic capacity (Chapter Twelve). Instead of being open to meeting and exploring the environment, the haptic function became protective, defending against receiving a sensation. We could call this an example of haptic dissociation, an inhibition in the ease of exchange with the world that can ensue after a trauma.

To explore the phenomenon further, Hubert and his colleagues chose to do a simple study of the Unbendable Arm using electromyography (EMG).[2] The publication process took years and eventually the study was published in 2001 in an Italian journal, *Manuale di Psiconcologia* (Godard *et al.*, 2001). The study included clinical observation and an EMG component looking into the mechanism behind what they had observed in breast cancer patients. Hubert had devised an experiment to see what was actually going on physiologically in the Unbendable Arm exercise. In tai chi classes, the change in strength is accounted for as an increase in qi flow. That is as far as it goes. But Hubert wanted to know what was different at the physiological level. By understanding the underlying mechanism, the phenomenon goes from being a magic trick to something I can deliberately apply in other situations.

In this case, the study was done on healthy subjects who were asked to keep their arm extended against resistance in three tests with slightly different conditions. In the first test, subjects were asked to keep the arm straight against resistance. In this case, the EMG results showed that both biceps and triceps contracted. In other words, the subject inadvertently helped the examiner bend the arm.

In the second test, subjects were asked to "imagine that your fingers lengthen out to reach the wall of the room," or "that your fingers emit a beam of light that reaches the wall." In most cases, both subject and opponent experienced the arm as stronger. Like Ramona, the subject reported feeling it was easier to keep the arm extended against resistance while using this visualization. The opponent reported feeling it was harder, if not impossible, to bend the arm. According to the EMG, in this case only the triceps fired. The perceived increase in strength could be accounted for by the lack of activity in the antagonist (biceps).

In the third test, the subjects were asked to do the same as in test 2, but during the exercise another doctor would cross the subject's visual field ("the aiming field")—essentially, they would walk through the background during the exercise. At the exact moment that the doctor passed through the imagined beam of light, the subjects' biceps again registered activity (Godard *et al.*, 2001, pp.878–879).

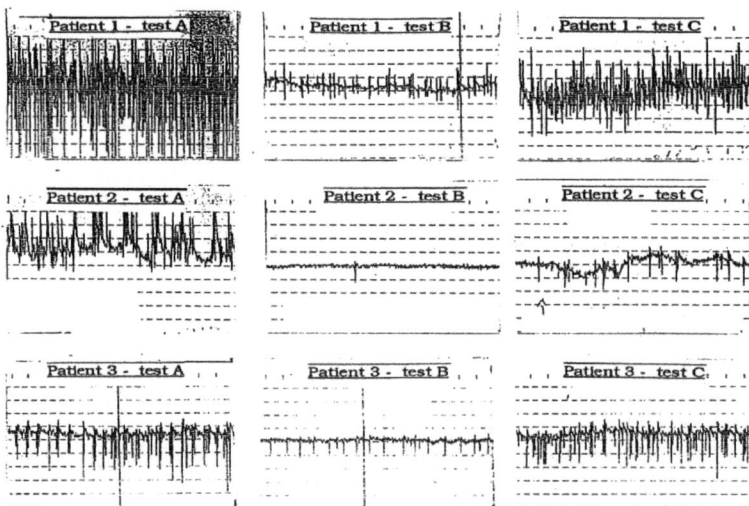

EMG Results, Biceps (Antagonist) Activity

How do we account for these results and what implications might they suggest? On an experiential level, connecting with our surroundings through our imagination seems to help us feel more secure. We become stronger with less effort—the feeling of effortless action. The study also suggests that we can go one step further to understand the physiological mechanism that is behind the effect. In the first test, what makes the subject's biceps contract when it goes against their conscious intention to keep their arm extended? In the second test, how does a change in perception, in how the subjects relate to the surrounding space, result in a change in motor pattern?

The authors of the study attribute the results of the Unbendable Arm experiments to changes in the gamma motor neuron firing pattern.[3] Simply put, alpha motor neurons fire in an all-or-none way when we give a voluntary command—"pick up the chair," for example. But the gamma motor neurons can modulate the activity of the alpha motor neurons. Considered together, the gamma neurons make up a system of their own, the fusimotor system, that relates muscle tone, fine motor coordination, emotional response, and orientation to the world (Ribot-Ciscar *et al.*, 2000, p.271).

The researchers suggest that the gamma system's activity provides a measurable parameter for studying the relationship of these complex activities. What appear to be changes in motor coordination and strength are the result of perceptual changes, a change in what we are imagining. The perceptual changes are not about the feeling inside the body: they are about the potential of action in the surrounding space. Physiologically, the changes in the contraction pattern of the muscles observed in the three tests correlate with a change in gamma firing. In the first test, the confrontational situation increases arousal; this fires the gamma neurons and leads to a contraction in the antagonist to the movement. But in the second test, in the same confrontational situation, when the subject's attention is directed to appropriate ex-proprioceptive information, the unnecessary gamma firing ceases. Gamma motor activity gives a neurological explanation for the results of the Unbendable Arm study, and for what may be happening when we experience ease in movement, effortless action, for ourselves.

From the first day of studying with Hubert, the image he painted of the body included the surroundings. In each workshop over the many years of working together, we considered the implications of our intertwining from a different angle and using different embodiments to experience it ourselves. Although most of us have probably convinced ourselves by adulthood that there is "me inside" in contrast to "out there," developmentally and in the present moment body and space are not two separate things. As Dr. Pierre Bonnier suggested in his book *L'Orientation* (1900), we can't perceive something (including ourselves) without perceiving some*where*.

Hubert would remind us that the surrounding space is always an action space for a baby or for an adult. We don't see the shape of the chair: we see the biomechanical actions that are associated with it. As Hubert mentioned in his 2009 talk in Montreux, that is why researchers like Gallese, Paillard, and others abandoned the term "body schema" in favor of adopting the term "action space." These scientists stopped using terms that imply a separation in favor of integrated terms like "body-in-space" or "embodied space." This change in terms also impacts how we work as practitioners with our clients.

CASE STUDY

Now that you have an inkling of the physiological mechanisms behind our sense of space, let's look at how we work with our sense of space in practice. The three sessions with a client I will call "Gracie" described below illustrate the power of understanding "body" as a reflection of a habit of orientation. Certain actions and perceptions follow from our choice, even impacting what we call emotion.

Gracie is referred by a colleague. When she comes into the room for her first session, she exclaims immediately at the great view and walks over to look out of the big windows that make up half the wall space of the office. Looking down from the eighth floor onto the roofs and streets of Cambridge below us, she says, "I live in the neighborhood. It's so interesting to see it from this perspective." She remarks on the clock in the City Hall tower that we can see directly in the center of the view.

I'm listening and picking up on the clues. Although the view often gets attention, this is not true for everyone. Certainly, not everyone goes right over to the windows to look straight down. Some people's attention is focused on me, or they may be preoccupied, in their own world, as they walk in the door. Others may see the view and wonder aloud if they are visible to all of Boston—a completely different response—or express some fear at the height. The various reactions to a wall of windows can be a revealing detail, something of a perceptual Rorschach. It can be a clue to how a person occupies the space.

Gracie's build is wiry, no extra padding, not muscle-bound, and yet there is a stiffness in her movement. She is verbal and expressive. She tells me that she meditates and has a long-standing yoga practice. She seems to have a lot of perspective on her internal processes. She tells me that she is an avid runner, so much so that she doesn't like to stop running outside even in the icy New England winters. She has even tried running in the snow with Yak Traks—an ice traction device that you pull on over your shoe—and she thinks that may be how she hurt her ankle to begin with.

She is pushing herself to sing in public ceremonies, but she experiences enormous anxiety in preparation for these events. Yet it is something she knows she wants to pursue.

On the one hand, she tells me how much she loves to get out there and run. Get outside, be active. But also, she talks about anxiety, in singing and in other situations in her life. When she walks around the room, I see another clue: the instability in her ankles, wobbling at each step. Maybe that makes her in a hurry to get off them. Although she's not literally running now, she still has forward momentum in her upper body that shifts the weight so that she leans forward, like Giacometti's "Walking Man" (Guggenheim Bilbao Museum, n.d.). [Figure 9] The weight of her trunk falls in front of her center of gravity—G' anterior.[4] She is picking up on and using signals from her inner ear as she runs, so she doesn't need the ground so much for that action.

These little clues show me what part of the space she picks up on perceptually—what she is used to paying attention to. She habitually picks up on the exteroceptive space, outside herself first; she chooses space more than ground as her primary orientation, using the information from her inner ear more than sensations from the ground into the feet. Gracie's "body" reveals her preferred actions: to run, to move forward, to feel light. As practitioners, when we get past seeing the symptoms in isolation, or focusing on one joint at a time, "body" becomes an expression of possible actions. One of Hubert's often-repeated expressions is "Posture is the potential of action."

Gracie already has a yoga practice, so at the end of the first session, I suggest that instead of doing balance poses in her usual way during the week ahead, she spend time in her practice focusing on the very beginning of the pose, when the weight is just shifting onto one foot. If Gracie practices in her usual way, she will be likely to skip this step. She would be reinforcing her usual tensions. To practice at this subtler level, taking the time to bear the weight on one foot, sensing the floor, will help increase her stability. It will give time for the muscles in the soles of the feet to do their sensory work, while the inner ear does its job of helping with balance. The exercise will not merely develop muscular strength at the ankles; it will help feed information through the nervous system that will lead to better stability. Hubert sometimes calls the action of the foot sensing the floor as the weight shifts "activating the suction cups," after an image he gleaned from tai chi.

In this first meeting with Gracie, my goal is to open up possibilities in how she orients in space. I am using body-reading skills as I let her words and actions show me her postural and perceptual preferences. Although in the hands-on part of the session, I may address "ownership" or interoceptive experience, the emphasis is on the action space. Her homework—to activate the suction cups of her feet—starts with the very beginning of the movement in order to reach her pre-movement, her perceptual choices.

Figure 9: "Walking Man"

Session two: The map is not the territory

When Gracie comes in the next week for her second session, we continue to explore what will help bring more of the "substratum," the ground and her sense of weight, into her perceptual repertoire.

She had officiated at a funeral and worked with the anxiety successfully, though still wishing it wasn't quite so difficult. She quotes another practitioner who told her that for animals, to stand up is to be eaten, to become prey. She offers this interpretation as a provisional explanation for her fear and anxiety.

Her comment reverberates in me. There is a tone to the statement, maybe something too defining.

She is referring to an important conceptual framework that reminds us that our nervous system has evolved over many millions of years. Our nervous system is of the fight-or-flight variety, and sometimes we can feel like the predator, but more likely like the prey. In that case, the organism takes over and prepares to fight or flee.

"The fear I am feeling is because the organism-that-is-me thinks I'm about to be devoured when I stand up in front of a group." This could be a useful framework in which she doesn't have to feel bad about her anxiety, and instead can see her personal anxiety in the context of her organism, her body as an animal. But it's only one point of view, one image. One map.

The downside is that it could also lock her into the experience. "Of course I'm going to feel anxious," she might assume, "because the organism-that-is-me feels like prey." This is an explanation, not an experience. I worry that her current explanation could prevent her from looking into her own experience more deeply. Knowing instead of not-knowing. Not-knowing is being open to the possibilities her anxiety may reveal. Maybe we shouldn't take for granted that this provisional explanation tells the whole story of her anxiety. The metaphor she has adopted is just one way of imagining the situation. My impulse, before I really have time to think, is to offer another image.

I say: "Metaphors are like shoes: you need more than one pair." I say: "What about a herd: the animal that hears the sound first picks up its head and that's a cue for all the other animals. It's information transmission, communication, sharing information." This is a different story, a different metaphor through which to imagine what it means to stand up and be seen.

She tells me that image better fits her singing in public. She thinks of herself in that context as sharing something with the audience, touching them. Changing the metaphor lets her reframe the situation for herself. Perhaps the anxiety is not inevitable after all.

Dr. Rolf liked to quote Alfred Korzybski's saying "A map is not the territory" (Korzybski, 1933, p.750). The situation, the territory, presents much more information, many more possibilities than any one metaphor can capture. The map is a simplification that can be useful for navigating a territory. But there can be many maps: for instance, for the US, there is a map showing the human/society-made shapes of the states, the boundary lines. But there could also be an "earth-centric" map, one that shows mountains and rivers and geology. Each map describes aspects of the territory, but the territory presents many options, as yet undiscovered. Hubert's model connecting the habits embedded in the body's structure with the habits embedded in the domains of perception, coordination, and meaning (Part II) helps me recognize the power of the symbolic when it arises in a session such as this. Some of the work that leads to a change in movement is a change in metaphor. This is as important for changing movement patterns as any of the other domains.

Session two continued: *Passaggio*

Picking up from where we had left off the previous week, Gracie takes a walk around the room. I suggest just slowing down so that she has a little more time to pick up sensory information from the ground through her feet, and so that her whole system can get used to organizing balancing and walking in a new way.

We slow down even more to notice the process of weight transfer from the back foot to front foot that occurs with each step: there is a lot going on for a human being in what might seem like a very simple act. In particular, this is the moment in the step when both feet can be on the ground at the same time. The front foot has landed, but the weight isn't committed to it just yet. In this moment, one can still go back or keep going forwards.

To have this option in walking does not go without saying. For Gracie, her forward momentum style and her running practice don't lead to taking much time in that moment, both feet on the ground, options open.

As we explore the phenomenon together, Gracie says, "Oh, that's like a *passaggio*." She goes on to explain that in singing, when the vocal register transitions from chest voice to head voice, it is often called a break in the voice. Singers tend to skip over the break, when what works better is to slow down and stay with the moment so that it can become smooth. She likens the way she feels in slow walking with the "break" where she notices the instability in her ankle and is tempted to go faster over that transition moment.

I am delighted! In many years of working with this movement and many different people's experiences and ways of expressing them, this is the first time I have heard this particular association. It is entirely Gracie's own. With this insight, she finds her own way to "make sense": to begin to change her quality of perception through language and movement practices that have the potential to open up new possible actions. Through her analogy, her own magic words, she will have access to a shift: to go from her usual "get off my feet" style to paying attention to the subtlety of weight transfer. Using this image/feeling/analogy between our sessions will help anchor a new option: to pay attention to the sensations involved in transferring weight, each step. By doing this activity throughout the week between our sessions, she will be practicing a new habit of perception and changing her brain's map.

In the voice, Gracie understands the value and importance of *passaggio*, so that, too, can be transferred over to the value of exploring another aspect of walking aside from the one she already knows.

Gracie's second session shows again how habits are embedded at multiple levels. They are habits of perception (the sensory/perceptual information I am picking up), coordination (how do I organize this movement?), orientation (what information and coordination am I using to not fall over while I'm doing other things?); and meaning (all the associations I have with this feeling, movement, coordination). She can use the symbol of a *passaggio* to shift her perceptual attention and take the time to feel the ground. This will help change her walking pattern—her coordination—to give her more push-off and less tension, all the while strengthening her ankles because she is using the musculature more effectively. All these levels are included in changing a movement pattern and are available for us to work with for ourselves and with our clients. This is the framework I learned from Hubert over the many years of study.

Some of the insights I experienced for myself through embodiment in workshops and sessions have stayed with me for years. Each one is a "breakthrough"—breaking through the unconscious habit pattern, providing an opportunity for a new experience.

Session three

When Gracie comes in for her third session, she sits down in the chair across from me. We talk about how the past week's practices have gone. She tells me that she has been enjoying the slow walk, when she is feeling the ground. We talk about potential actions, how they are different when you are getting vestibular information compared to picking up cues from the ground. The felt presence of ground makes new options available.

"Let's try something that will help you experience what I am talking about," I say. The week before I had used this experiment in a workshop I taught at the Boston Conservatory based on a memorable exercise Hubert had us do 20 years before.

In the large, bare studio, I ask the students to sit on chairs facing their partner who is several yards away, also sitting on a chair. I demonstrate with the director of the program, Debi. We get up from the chair using one or the other strategy (vestibular versus ground). We note our own experience, and the students observe the theatre—what they see happening between us.

With the vestibular strategy, when we both choose to focus on the sensation of orienting from the head, through our senses or sense of the room, we both move lightly, freely going to greet the other person.

But when we both choose the sense of the ground, tuning in to the sensations (information) between our feet and the ground, as we stand up, neither of us goes anywhere! There is no desire to go, to move forward. Both of us just stand where we are, feeling the ground.

The students laugh at the visible expression of "standing our ground" and how the obvious difference in the "story" is shown by the two different strategies.

The students then tried out the experiment with their partners. They reported feeling very involved with the other person when they used sky orientation, and much less so with the ground, perhaps even feeling that they did not care about the other person. They also reported their preferences: some felt comfortable with one strategy but clearly not with the other.

In my office, Gracie and I try out a similar experiment. When she stands up in her usual way, she seems to be already running, almost running into me. There is a slight impression that she is out of control. This might be true for any one of us: without the capacity to rest into the ground, there is no option to stay where we are. In just standing, there is already forward momentum.

Gracie notices how her pre-movement—the perceptual habit of taking in only a certain part of the environment—interacts with her self-report of anxiety. She mentions the social anxiety that she experiences even when she is talking to her very kind boss, and then puts it together for herself: Maybe the action the body is primed for is bringing the anxiety.

This is William James's point in the essay "What Is an Emotion?" when he asked (my paraphrase): "Do we run from the bear because we are afraid, or do we feel afraid because we run?" (James, 1884, p.190). For Gracie, the patterned movements, the ones that make her need to move, to run, to get out, are one aspect of the nervous system: flight. The physical sensations are giving her the message that there is something to fear. But when she tunes in to the information beneath her feet, to the way the ground feels in the present moment, then her nervous system receives different information: okay to stay here. New actions become possible for her when the perception of the ground is selected.

With Gracie, tuning into the space behind her—the backfield—also allows her to have a different feeling when approaching me. Gracie calls it "broadening."

Through the sessions we did together, Gracie learned to have a choice in terms of her perceptions, her postures, and her actions. She found a relationship to new sources of support the environment affords: the ground under her feet and the balance of her sense of space to include behind her as well as in front gave her more ways to find stability, which led to more options in her behavior—more potential actions. The process also led to diminished anxiety.

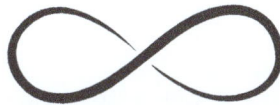

∞

The old joke is that a stopped clock is right twice a day. Posture shows the potential of action, and the action has to suit the context. If we don't have a range of possible actions, if we are inadvertently stuck in one preference, then we are liable to find ourselves uncomfortable in certain situations. We need to direct our attention to new perceptions and new ways of imagining to develop a range of new actions. We have much more choice in these matters than we tend to exercise.

Coming back to Dr. Rolf's maxim "If you want a different conclusion, start with a different premise" (Feitis, 1978, p.42), how does it apply here? With a range of terms like ownership and agency, and action space which includes the surroundings, we can reimagine somatic practice. As practitioners, we can be more specific about the domain and the intention of a session. Opening our imagination of somatic practice allows us to recognize the territory—what part of the landscape of embodiment we find ourselves in at a given moment in a session so we can creatively respond.

In our personal somatic practice—when we use forms in tai chi or yoga, for example—we can clarify our intention: we can vary our pre-movements by choosing different starting points for orientation—starting from the earth, or letting go, or feeling the surrounding space, to name only a few—and different ways of imagining as we have explored in Part IV.

With such a rich range of possibilities, what keeps us repeating movement patterns or pre-movements that don't serve us? Why don't we use our choices? One reason is that our perceptual patterns start before our memory is fully formed. Part V will go into more depth about developmental processes, and how we access change as adults.

PART V

BECOMING

CHAPTER SEVENTEEN

Secure Body

NOTHING TO DEFEND

It wasn't until I was standing in front of Petró that I realized that something was dramatically different.

2013. We were in Spain at the first in a new workshop series taking place at a luxurious beachside resort. Hubert liked to be warm. It was a long trip from Boston to Conil de la Frontera, with its houses all painted white to keep as cool as possible during the hot summer—a new location for me, but familiar for the Europeans. It was the end of September, pleasant but not sweltering. We came from near and far—as far as the U.S. and Brazil and as close as a nearby town in southern Spain—to green lawns dotted with chairs and loungers, multiple swimming pools, hot tubs in and out of doors, with two meals a day at the grand hotel buffet and the ocean just a quick walk across the road.

It was Wednesday, the third of our days together. The next day would be a day off. From the grand ballroom, with its adobe-tiled floors and large windows, we could hear the clanks and tinkling of dishes and silverware. Waiters and waitresses called out to each other in Spanish from the large patio next door. An ocean breeze wafted into the room. It was hot, and the windows and doors were wide open, the floor-to-ceiling curtains drawn to shield us from the sun's rays.

We sat on chairs arranged in a circle. As usual, Hubert started each day of the workshop introducing an idea, creating a conceptual framework for the work we would be doing in movement later or while exchanging sessions. This day, Hubert brought us back to the four foundational articulations: four dimensions of movement that need both connection and the capacity to be distinct, to separate (see Articulation in Chapter Two): the capacity to separate top and bottom, front and back, and side to side, and the capacity for our gaze to zoom out and zoom in. Hubert chose the term "foundational" specifically to avoid reiterating the assumption, common in developmental thinking, that we all go through the same *fundamental* stages or processes.[1] Putting that developmental perspective aside, our foundations are a temporal issue, where we have come from, each one of us in our own journey. Each time we use the term "foundational," we are trying to emphasize the importance of each individual's process and context instead of artificial standards that are supposed to apply uniformly.

The foundational articulations, Hubert had been reminding us, were not necessarily between the literal bones at all. He said that two of the most important articulations for good organization in gravity and free movement came from the capacity to separate top and bottom, and front and back. Separating top and bottom could be interpreted as allowing the chest and pelvis to let go of each other, but also beyond the flesh, allowing a sense of the sky and the ground, heaven and earth. As we saw in Chapter Eight, our physiology supports two opposing directions: for top and bottom, the vestibular system orients the head, and the feet orient the pelvis and bottom half of the body. Years before, we had worked with pushing the chair to evoke a sense of front and back, keeping our own weight centered while allowing the arms to go with the chair.

Today's exercise, this meditation based on Gerda Alexander's work Eutony,[2] was to help us experience the spine as an axis that could give a feeling of support from behind, which would leave the ribs free to move. Through this approach, Hubert suggested, we could affect the breath indirectly by creating a sense of support that would leave the body with breathing room. Hubert also reminded us that a good body image may not need detailed anatomical reference points for movement: the vectors described by top and bottom, front and back may be even more effective than knowing all the names of bones and muscles. This exercise was as much for the phenomenological body—the body as lived—as for the literal flesh.

Hubert demonstrated a movement exploration with one of the students, and then invited us to try it for ourselves. He gave us a choice to work with a partner or alone, allowing each of us to follow our own path. I worked by myself, as it's often easier for me to explore on my own without the complication of someone else's input. I lay on a yoga mat with a wooden stick running the length of my spine, from just below my neck almost to my hips.

Lying on the yoga mat with the stick beneath me, I found a resting place in the stick/spine and felt the ribs become free. Returning my attention to the spine, the breastbone was free to settle, to surrender to gravity. It was almost a meditation on inviting the stick to come in, to come up and become part of my spine. Non-doing: my only job was to put my attention on specific perceptions, the stick as it made its impression, the joyous freedom of the breath unfettered.

To finish, I took a moment as Hubert directed us to feel the ribs move in a chest breath, and then to imagine the lungs in the pelvis, and let the breath happen there. It could be called a belly breath, but when that more common image is invoked, it often brings with it an inadvertent tension, a small fear. Something contracts between the chest and pelvis (top-bottom) instead of letting go. With the image of the lungs in the pelvis, there is no trying, just imagining and experiencing.

Doing the exercise lying down felt pleasant but not particularly vivid, a chance to make contact with the stick and the floor, to feel the movement of the breath. To end the exercise, Hubert said, "And now you will face each other, and you will offer the stick of wood."

Standing in front of Petró after doing the exercise, I remember feeling the absence of weight on my chest. It was astounding: to stand in front of another person without my shield. At first, it felt so very vulnerable, so open, almost intolerable—and all we were doing was just standing across from each other.

After the first feeling of impossible openness, a glimmer arose: how funny it was to call this unprotected! Those habitual contractions, that shielding tension between the ribs and hips, did absolutely nothing to actually protect me in any way! What was it defending me from? How were the tensions protecting me? This moment in front of Petró was the real integration for me of the change in the movement pattern. Here was a bodily experience of being in a moment of relationship, of meeting another and not needing to defend, a moment of freedom from the usual defensive pattern, the character knot. It made room to notice that the previous contractions not only did not serve a real purpose, but that it was a relief to be free of them. It was a remarkable transformation. Through my experience lying on the stick, an axis had emerged, a new form of support that didn't require my habitual tension in the chest. This led to a new possibility of standing in relation to another person.

An experience such as this stays with us. Once a pattern is perceived, it becomes accessible. The flash of consciousness transforms the unconscious action into something we can work with. Feeling how we create our experiences, how our experiences emerge from small, unconscious habits of perception, allows new possibilities to emerge.

Then I offered the stick to Petró. There was no resistance to letting go of the stick, no grasping, no hesitation in offering it.

I was aware at that moment of the evolution that had happened over the years of working with Hubert. I can remember another class, long ago, when having my own "standing" (coming to stand with the new feeling of my own center in front of another student) felt distinctly like not giving a damn about the other person. Back then, I realized in a flash that I had somehow associated "caring" with a vague feeling of not quite being in balance—how dangerous! At that time, my first impression when I was over my own feet, free to move in any direction, was that it felt forbidden. To be neutral felt frightening, as if my life depended on being focused on someone else. Again, this is years ago, and yet it is still vivid. It sticks with me as a moment of "aha," through an embodied experience, a sudden revelation of a deep and perhaps very primal attitude that had been unconscious until then.

Hubert called this process perceiving "the secondary benefit" of a pattern, the way the pattern is serving me. Whatever I am doing to organize myself in gravity may not be the best way from a biomechanical point of view, and it is certainly not the only way, but for me and each one of us, those patterns of contraction have a purpose. They often keep us from feeling something uncomfortable or taboo. This is another example of the missing gesture we explored in Chapter Nine.

When there is a missing gesture, it can become a focal point. So much energy is going into not doing it that it shapes the potential of all the other actions. Potential because the inhibition interferes with our capacity to imagine. What we are trying to reclaim is the possibility, the imaginary, not necessarily to literally make the inhibited gesture. Of course, it's not dangerous in itself, or to anyone else perhaps, but for each one of us, meeting our psychomotor organization can feel a little threatening or exposing. There is a dimension of what we call posture that has come about from our earliest relationships with the people who surround us from our first day. Something of our past is with us in the present, expressed in a series of subconscious contractions that help us maintain our position. Strategies adopted much earlier in life, to manage in the context of that time, often live below the level of consciousness in the present. But in a flash, the story can be revealed, the strategies can be abandoned or modified, a world of possibilities can be revealed.

Before that moment, I felt the effects of the unconscious attitude in my relationships. I felt it as fear of attachment, fear of being engulfed by another person. As in my first experiences of Rolfing, the embodied flash went far beyond what I could say in words about feeling stuck in an emotional response pattern. It was a revelation of the underpinnings, the shaping that led to a persistent feeling, and, as such, was also a kind of liberation: in the instant of perceiving what I am doing, how I am doing it, other options become available, no matter what my infant or childhood patterns of relationship might have been. The insight of "what prevents me" is often imperceptible until we are standing in front of another person. It is in relationship that it becomes apparent.

These examples of moments of embodiment that did not feel like my usual way, the familiar *me*, have become reference points, something I can use to find my way. Because I understand the physical way I am creating a pattern, I can find a way out of the identity each time. People in psychotherapy will sometimes say, "I know what I'm doing but I can't help it." I think that's because the awareness is not an embodied experience. One way to describe the difference might be to distinguish intellectual understanding—a mental idea—from a perceptual understanding, which is inherently embodied.

When Hubert gathered us back together after the group had had a chance to explore the exercise, class members talked about their experiences and asked questions. To speak and listen to others about the variety of effects is important. Maybe it is in putting words to the experience that we take ownership of it. This was a common strategy in workshops and in sessions. Hubert said:

> Integration means finding the possibility of the new feeling/movement with another person; integration is being able to retrieve it without the teacher, and in our daily relationships. Maybe not all the time but having the possibility.

The words and concepts that Hubert provided helped me make the experience my own. They helped me find a way in, but without the embodiment the words would not have sufficed. Through embodiment *and* through words—the two ways of perceiving are essential. Words are symbols. The foundational articulations provide a rich set of symbols, a conceptual framework that includes our gravity organization. These concepts make available more complex perceptions about "body" than the posed corpses of Body Worlds where we started our journey of reimagining earlier in this book.

The process that had such a profound impact on me may affect someone else completely differently. You can't turn an exercise into a predictable formula to achieve a particular goal or meaning. You have to try it and find out what happens. When you work with the elements of how a person constructs a sense of self, a sense of space, you often stumble on important layers. Personally, that is what makes my own embodiment practice and the work with others continue to be riveting on a daily basis. There's no knowing exactly what will lead to a flash, but in the process of exploring the fundamentals of how we organize our uprightness, listening, and staying curious, it happens.

PHOROS

In Chandolin, years before, when Hubert first said jokingly, "You can't saw off the branch you are sitting on," he meant that you need to be able to find another source of support before you can let go of the one upon which you depend. It is true, literally and metaphorically. Since contexts are always changing, having more than one place to rest your weight is a crucial adaptability. That year in Spain, Hubert began to use a new term—*phoros*—in order to distinguish this movement phenomenon: to initiate movement by finding support that allows a separation, as when I gave the stick to Petró. As in the experience just described, the strategy we employ—our choice of "branch"—may go back a long way. Inevitably, how each one of us finds this foundational coordination—to let go into support before moving—has its origin in our first relationships, our earliest days before we have language to express ourselves. The pre-movements and associations we build up during this preverbal but foundational time of our development exist below the level of consciousness, yet are well practiced, present in each moment.

Let me give you an example: A former client visiting from out of town brings her eight-month-old baby to my office to introduce us. Lying on his back in the carrier, Cody's eyes are bright and curious. As soon as he is unbuckled, he reaches out to his mom with the familiarity of eight months of life. As she holds him up over her shoulder, he swivels around to explore the room, and me, the unfamiliar person. She sets him down on the floor, and he sits, Buddha-like, with a mostly bald head that seems to float in the air as if suspended or helium-filled. Legs easily fall into a supportive base, his bottom firmly settled on the floor. The ease with which he settles into the floor is an echo of the reception experienced in his mother's arms for the past months. From this well-supported resting, his top half can be relatively independent. With a clear sense of security, he can easily balance on one side or the other as he turns to follow us with his gaze. This child is a model of comfortable babyhood. He reflects a process of development that is at once physical and psycho-emotional: there is a sense of emotional and physical security that together allow for freedom of movement, a base that makes room for exploration.

We mostly don't remember this phase of our life, and yet even more than elementary school math skills form the basis for learning calculus later on, even more than learning to shape each letter leads to reading and writing, this eight-month-old baby is building on foundational skills he has already established in a close relationship with his mother. These building blocks shape all his movements, and in some ways establish relationship patterns in the physical sense of how he finds a place to rest, a sense of what supports him—colloquially, we could say "where he is coming from." In order to emphasize the importance of this elusive phenomenon, Hubert began to call the quality of finding support *phoros*, from the ancient Greek term for "carry" or "bear" (*pherein*, to be borne or carried) (Bullinger, 2010, p.11).

Foundational articulations

The simple scene of Cody I just described includes many of the elements that are involved in this early stage of development. The gesture of reaching for his mom shows the profound intimacy of eight months, the familiar and comfortable relationship, full of expectation. This gesture has already had a lot of practice time and reflects a complex coordination. Resting on his back, the child can feel enough support so that he can let his arm release in a reach. When the coordination of reaching is lacking at this stage of a baby's development, it's a red flag (Bullinger, 2010).

His mother holds him, orients him, and provides the supportive base for his visual exploration. His head knows which way is up already, but her support allows him to see much farther off than he could manage on his own. We don't usually think of vision as an articulation, but Hubert introduced "vergence," the capacity of the eyes to zoom in and out, as one of the four foundational articulations. It is based on the capacity of pupils to move towards each other and away from each other when we bring our eyes in and out of focus. Cody can coordinate movement and gaze as he swivels around to see me.

Hubert applied this fourth foundational articulation to all the senses, not just vision. It refers to our presence in the space through our sensory systems. The freedom to move between far and near, or broad and narrow perception, rather than being stuck either in a focal (What) or a peripheral (Where) position, affects the system of articulations as a whole. It describes how we inhabit space. We thus try to avoid creating a concept of a body that is separate from the landscape that is being constructed.

Sitting, Cody has his own base from the sensation of the floor under his seat when he sits upright. The base receiving support while the top moves seems like an obvious possibility, but when you start to look at adults, you see how often it has been lost. In adults, so often the chest and pelvis are not free from each other. Washboard abs, in fact, literally pull the chest onto the pelvis and vice versa. Body image is built at the expense of freedom of movement, freedom of expression, and curiosity.

Cody's vestibular support—the other side of the "base"—is reflected in a head that seems to float. He shows a clear capacity in both ways of sensing gravity. With these coordinations in place, he has developed a sense of an axis—a supportive scaffolding from his trunk, neck, and head—that goes far beyond the anatomical structures. Top to bottom, front to back, and then side to side as he balances on one sitting bone, these could be called the other three foundational articulations that allow movement. They free the baby from symmetrical, fetal postures, and let him be open to the stimulations, opportunities (affordances) of his environment.

With these capacities of movement in the gravitational field established at a good-enough level, the first thing Cody wants to do, given enough safety, is explore the environment.

No need for words for this boy—he is completely expressive without them. There is no "body" for this baby—there is curiosity, movement, emotion, expression, but no "head," "shoulders," and "knees." These words/concepts have yet to be introduced, for better or for worse. Instead, there is the experience of balancing (at least in the sitting position), of weighting and unweighting, a beginning of play with gravity. There is reaching and exploring. He may not be talking, but he is learning about physical reality, studying physics through his body—how the floor responds to his push. A lot of learning is going on here! He is learning through his interactions with his physical environment.

When he finds himself on all fours, he inadvertently moves away from his goal: his arms have more coordination and strength from the past months' movements than his legs, so pushing takes him backwards. But also, he is wearing soft-soled slippers that slide on the carpet and don't give him much purchase for forward momentum. It will soon come. Independent movement, crawling, standing, walking, and running are still before him, but the ground and sky of posture and tone have been prepared.

In our early infancy, emotion, the process of gaining independence, meeting the world, organizing perception, and organizing our movements are all happening together, in relation to each other. Later in life, we mostly forget this. It's as if we see a tree's branches against the sky without realizing that they grew from the trunk that is right in front of us, with its roots in the ground. Later in life, even with good will, it can be hard to change our behavior if we don't realize and work with its deep physical and perceptual underpinnings. This also explains why change in adulthood can be so challenging. Intellect alone does not reach the pre-verbal, developmental level. Movement, imagination, touch, and sensory awareness do. Hubert's concept of *phoros*—how we find support, how we can organize our weight to allow something else to let go—spotlights a foundational aspect of movement and development that we can work with ourselves.

PHORIC ACTIVITY

We spent time at the 2013 workshop in Spain exploring what Hubert meant by *phoros*, talking about it, and making sense of it for ourselves. To use a new word like *phoros* to describe a phenomenon runs the risk of creating confusion, but Hubert was masterful at tying together theory and practice.

When we arrived at the workshop space on Wednesday morning, the third day of the workshop, there was a drawing of two figures on the newsprint pad. The first was a sort of closed clamshell. In the second, the halves had been separated completely, one going up and the other down, with a red line connecting them. Hubert called this the "cursor," in the sense of a mobile element that can move at will, sliding between here and there.

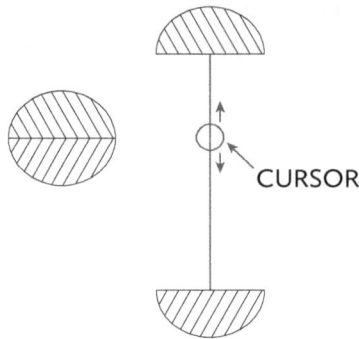

"When I say separation, or phoric activity," Hubert said, pointing to the diagram, "it's like going from the first diagram to the second. You create a gap, a separation between top and bottom. Then I can go this way"—Hubert rose from the chair, letting his upper body lead, and there was a sense that his lower half was still resting toward the ground. "Or this way," he said as he sat back down with the weight of his lower half leading him, while his chest seemed to still float for a moment. "This dynamic cannot happen if the two parts are glued together. The question of moving is not really about what moves," Hubert said. "It is about what doesn't move."

This is simple to say, but unexpectedly profound. In general, in movement, in dance or sports activity, we give the attention to the part that is moving, and not to the supporting side. Hubert went on, "I have to take the time to build what doesn't move, and then I can move. I can't move my leg if I am in my leg. I have to build a place where I am not my leg so that I can move my leg."

TRY THIS ✓

Try it now, sitting in your chair. Let your arm go up and feel what is tensing in your shoulders. Then bring in the phoric activity: instead of keeping the focus on your arm, come to rest in your trunk, let yourself rest in your pelvis, and then allow the separation of the arm.

The work, the attention, goes to the process that enables us to find another place to rest than in the arm. It could be by finding more support for the head, the neck, the spine—it is an activity created anew in each moment. This is the activity that will free the shoulder. Resting in another place and offering the arm.

This is what Hubert called phoric activity.

No map

One of the students asked if phoric activity was like remapping, creating a better map of the body. Hubert responded:

> Remapping implies that there is a map, and then we are creating another map. But here, there is *no* map. Because mapping already implies a theory of being—linked to a body schema. It comes with a whole philosophical point of view. Whereas phoric activity is constantly reinvented.

He went on:

> We're not talking about foundational movement as an ontological vision. In the beginning of the last century, there was an ontological idea of foundational movement, where they said that each baby develops in movement by doing the same stages in the same order. It's not like that. Movement develops in relationship to context.

He was standing at the easel, showing the lower half of the clamshell: "You will be here"—and then showing the upper half—"and you offer that to the world. This is me"—the lower half—"and my arm can go away. Or the opposite: I can be here, at the top, and let the other one go."

In French, the literal translation of "shaking hands" is "to give someone your hand." Hubert said, "When we shake hands, I give you my hand, but if I can't separate the hand from the rest of the body, then I can't give it." He demonstrated with a student, Simone:

> I can give my hand to the world, and I can accept Simone to come inside me when I shake her hand. It's not holding, it's huge hapticity. For her to do that, she has to be sitting on the chair—she is not the hand, not the arm, she is on her bottom on the chair.

Hubert's concept of phoric is the capacity to allow a separation within us. He said, "It's very important, because this—whichever one we let go—is like 'the Other.'" The two parts express a difference in status: one takes on the role of support. It expresses the continuity of a gravitational *self*. That frees the movement of the Other—which could be the other leg, the other arm, the body itself moving. In that moment, from the point of view of support, I let go of what is *me*. Hubert noted that joint problems are often a result of the lack of clarity about this topology.

TRY THIS

In sitting, in the previous example, we let the arm go away—into abduction—moving away from the midline. This time, start on the floor. With your hand on the floor, the abduction slides the body away from the arm. How do you allow yourself to "become" your arm, to let the body be free to slide?

Hubert said:

> This is something we are constantly creating. It's an articulation but beyond the bone level, on another level. We are creating a separation. There's a lot of philosophy behind this. Inside me, I need to be able to divide myself into pieces. There is often resistance to letting the body shift like this. Psychologically, we fear dismemberment. To be able to move, we need to be able to dismember. We need to be able to shift back and forth between (1) being in the arm and letting the body go away, and (2) staying in the body and letting the arm go away.

Dismemberment is a powerful image! So much of our lives we are "trying to keep it together." We fear chaos, things falling apart. What Hubert was pointing us towards with his language was a remarkable activity that we could practice: instead of needing to cling to one support with which we identified, we could allow our support to vary in response to the situation.

Phoros can seem deeply philosophical, but it is also a practical movement skill. For example, when the hand is active without the forearm muscles contracting, there is a separation of the activity of short and long flexors in the forearm and hand. They do not automatically have to work at the same time. The capacity of short and long flexors to keep some independence can allow a lot more freedom of movement in the wrist than if they are always glued together. But in another context—for instance, if lifting a heavy load or stopping something from falling—we would want them to work together. We want to have options in our motor and perceptual system to allow us to meet each situation.

Pushing the chair after 25 years

Hubert reminded us of non-doing, the concept in Chinese philosophy. He showed again the many ways to move a chair—how we can push it with a concentric compressive movement, or instead, if we want the chair to slide, we can create a gap. Doing it the first way compresses the articulation, and doing it the other way decompresses. This is *wei wu wei*—action without action—of moving the chair. It may be invisible from the outside, but it is a completely different process. "The chair is not me anymore, my arm is not me. It's not visible—there is something that happens inside you when you shift."

This brought me back to years ago when we first did this exercise in Philadelphia. Pushing the chair (Chapter Two), a familiar exercise, yet with this new term—*phoros*, phoric activity—there was an increasingly refined description of what was involved. It was an experience for me now, a long way from "tonic function" and "two directions." We need this kind of rich language to describe embodiment and its relationship to sense of self, cultivating a different idea of what self/Other means through bodily experience connected to concepts and language. This is yet another "articulation," a way of describing a surprising phenomenon that allows us to see it, to feel it, and to communicate about it.

BACKING

When the group gathered again after the exploration, we shared our experiences. Then Hubert said, "Phoric activity is the capacity to find multiple possibilities of support—to find support in a multitude of ways."

> You can't saw off the branch you are sitting on. The holding is not a tissue problem, a lesion. The problem arises when I cannot allow the separation of two parts of my body, giving each one its own status: one establishes support while the other engages with the world. If you sit on the branch of the tree, you cannot saw it off. Something in you will resist. That is what I would call a "phoric limitation." You have to sit on another branch.

In gesture, the imaginary appears in our ability to create many articulations through these changes in status—the capacity to allow the locus of support to vary and to allow the separation between different parts of the body. Just so, the foundational articulations play between the directions in space, earth, and sky, expanding into one part of the kinesphere, then another, like in our meditation with the colored balls (Chapter Fifteen). In sitting, when we put the weight on one sitting bone (ischial tuberosity), so the other one can move; or we allow the gaze to change depending on the circumstances—we are constantly reimagining what is "me" and what is moving.

Hubert pointed out that in each approach to movement, there would be a concept pointing to this phoric activity and practices related to it.

Tai chi

In the saying from tai chi, for example: *Han xiong, ba bei*—the chest relaxes while the spine lengthens.[3] This saying doesn't describe a specific anatomical joint but can be experienced as a kind of separation: the front roots while the back expands into the world. In practice, this change of support and freedom to let go can happen in a myriad of ways—within a limb, one side with the other, front and back, up and down, et cetera. In tai chi, there is also the idea of filling and emptying, or substantial and insubstantial: as you move, one limb fills as the weight is transferred to it and the other empties. We give the weight to one limb to free the other to be light—insubstantial—so it can move easily. Even walking is the process of loading one limb and unloading the other. The familiar metaphor to follow the qi helps free us from too much effort. The qi is moving, not me—not my doing.

Yoga

For an example from yoga, Hubert described the "bandha." Translated as link, connection, or sometimes as lock, the bandhas are strategic zones at the neck (*jālandhara bandha*), the pelvis (*mūla bandha*), and the respiratory diaphragm (*uddīyāna bandha*). He said: "The bandha bring together—connect, in French *relier*—and separate at the same time. It's a meeting place as well as a boundary, a separation; a differentiation and a meeting." Michel Alibert, yoga teacher and colleague of Hubert's, writes: "To practice 'bandha' is not first to do something, but first to perceive a link and work for this and with this" (Alibert, 2014, p.65).[4] Instead of using muscular contraction to lock these areas, Alibert suggests a more delicate way of using the bandha. The spine connects all three areas. The sense of support (*phoros*) can move between the spine in the back, the lower part of transversus abdominis in the front, and the longus colli muscle in the front of the neck. With a sense of two directions for the spine elicited at the root/pelvis and neck, engaging *uddīyāna bandha* allows the diaphragm to fully release in exhaling. The breath can be supported in a multitude of ways in inhaling and exhaling rather than rigidifying into an idea of one correct way to breathe.

Pilates

In Pilates, as well, we can use the Reformer (Pilates machine) in a way that invites us to keep changing the fixed point and letting different parts lead out into space. As our hands meet the bar and feet meet the platform, we can rest into those areas while head or tail reaches into space. Or different parts of the feet—under the toes, the arch, the heels—can be the point of contact. Hubert called this "esoteric or metaphysical Pilates." It results from taking a different attitude: if we just focus on the "powerhouse," we can miss out on the phoric aspect.

He went on:

> Or you can imagine a meditation on the theme of *phoros*. It's a meditation of creating a gap, to elicit a gap, a separation in the body. Even in talking you are giving your voice. I can give my front and it's not confusing because there is a back. When I'm talking there is nothing that prevents the vocal cords' vibration, and the expressive activity.

This idea or feeling of backing gives us the possibility of giving freedom to the front.

Hubert said:

> It's impossible to give something to somebody if you don't have front/back separation. You cannot give, you can even not forgive. The building of the phoric is necessary to be able to give a gift. Even words are an offering. You can't do it if you don't have a place in your body that you are secure, where you can stay.

The idea of *phoros* also applies when we work with someone as a practitioner. We can take the time to ask the person to find a place to rest other than the place we are seeking movement, and we can find the support that allows our own hand to follow the person.

Hubert described this process in more detail:

> It's so important when I work with someone that I am not in my arm and

my hand. I create a gap with my hand in such a way that my hand is given to the client, and I'm not that hand. If I can find this capacity, the client will be capable of doing it too, to give his leg, and not be afraid. Then it's as if there are three people: there is the client, there is me, and there is a third body that is made of the leg of the client and my arm. It may seem philosophical, but it is very concrete for the joints.

Hubert told us that, as with *haptos*, he chose to give a name, *phoros*, to this phenomenon to call attention to it. The practice of lying on the stick was a chance to practice introducing the "Other" into us, so there could be what he called "an elasticity," a psychological welcome. Not cutting the Other, but to keep on including the Other in your space.

What Hubert called "phoric capacity," the skill we were practicing in this workshop, enables us to keep our boundary while being open to an Other. Core activity, in the sense of how we keep our balance or find stability, can be elicited from the hand, the feet, head, eyes, depending on the way we meet the world. Are we in fusion, grasping, overly attached? Pushing away, distancing? Or can we find a comfortable adaptability? Hubert said, "I can go away, and still even if I am far away, I am still in intimacy with you."

EMBODIMENT: A MEDITATION ON BREATH

To end the day, we applied the idea of *phoros* to the breath, following from the first embodiment practice described at the beginning of the chapter.

Let's follow this embodiment, starting from sitting. Since it is a meditation, you may want to record it or read one instruction and try it before going on to the next one. The pacing matters, so take your time.

Feel the weight of the spine resting back against the chair.

Being attentive to our own ease in gravity, how are we sitting, how are we feeling the weight of the body resting—to make room for the movement of the breath? We can't work with the breath if there isn't some feeling of this gravity relationship.

Resting on the spine, let yourself feel a big space opening before you. Offer yourself a "spatial legitimacy," an infinite universe in front of you that is an attractor for the ribs.

This is the most important: differentiating the column (the sense of an axis, not the material spine) and the surrounding space.

Going from one to the other: sometimes come back to the exhale, the weight of the spine; sometimes to the opening of the space.

You aren't responsible for the breath, but for having a spine and the space opening.

The space could be an acoustic space—the space of sounds—or a visual space—they are different.

This isn't working on the breath; it's on the pre-movement of the breath, the preparation.

How do you imagine the space? Imagining the infinite? Open rather than infinite?

Then there is the olfactory space—catching a smell from a passing breeze—a whiff of forest, of pine? This can open the top cervical vertebra.

A tactile space: each pore of the skin, everywhere, will open to the cool, fresh air stimulating each pore and then the heat inside as I come back to the exhalation.

The breath depends on your imagination, the way you construct the surrounding space.

Then how do we go from one to the other? The pre-movement of inspiration: the sense of the spine and of the horizon, infinite, auditory, tactile, olfactory...

And because of the pre-movement, the exhale begins before inhaling is completely finished.

There is no break between inhale and exhale.

At the end of exhaling, in contrast, we can rest with the weight, until something inspires me—it's the invention of the space.

In normal breathing, like a wave on the beach, as the water comes up on the sand, there is already something returning to the ocean. The pre-movement of exhaling begins before the end of the inhale.

When we try to control our breath, there is an emotional quality. It can feel almost like the spine has moved to the front; the backing is lost.

The sternum doesn't go up and down with the breath in upright posture but moves horizontally.

It's as if every exhalation you faint; there is a surrender. Not closing in the front, but just "expiring"...letting go...dying...

Many people will shorten in front to exhale, in order to control the expression of emotion, so it is not so easy to let go.

You can do this against the wall to give support to the place that closes.

Imagine a sail that is lifting and then sinking instead of the sail being pulled back down. The Patanjali sutra says, "Prana flies on the wings of a great bird." That's the feeling.

The symbolic construction of space is primary in shaping the body.

If you are having trouble organizing the breath, stop working with the breath and go back to the pre-movements—the spine, the cobra, opening the space, but without reference to the breath.

Then we stand up from our chairs, going to encounter another with the immensity of space, resting on the spine.

CHAPTER EIGHTEEN

Becoming

As I explored earlier in the scene with Cody, and as I found in my own experience, the preverbal world of the infant still lives in me, in us. We learn to move in a world with a specific gravity and particular people. Although during early infancy, memory in its current understanding is not yet formed, formative experiences are occurring. On some level, in adulthood, each of us is still with that baby.

Under Hubert's influence, my curiosity about babies led me to Daniel Stern's (1934–2012) wonderful book, *The Interpersonal World of the Infant* (1985), and the fascinating research into the question "What do infants know?" Stern was both a psychoanalyst and a specialist in child development. In the introduction to his book, he recounts how his two specializations influenced his research. As a developmental psychologist, he knew that memory forms only later in a child's life, but in the context of psychoanalysis, his patients reported having a sense of their own infant experience. How to reconcile these two realities?

I could relate to this question. As I mentioned to Benjamin in his session (Chapter Thirteen), years ago I had vivid dreams about a baby with no skin—a gripping image for me. Without skin, the dream baby had no way to protect herself from overwhelming sensation. I had wondered about my own experience as an infant. I had always heard how much crying I did as a baby. My father's handwriting attests to it on page after page of the baby book that documents my first year: three months, "she cries"; four months, "she still cries"; seven months, eight months, ten months, and finally, 18 months, "she cries because she likes to cry." Clearly it made an impact on him! Why was that baby crying? The wordless tears evoked by my first Rolfing sessions seemed to well up from a part of me that did not speak any other language. Was that the infant's experience? How might it still be with me today?

Daniel Stern's research and Hubert's perspective on the development of perception and movement organization in infancy helped me imagine—to really get a feel for—what this baby might have been experiencing. I keep the infant perspective in mind even when working with adults. The basis of tone arises in the preverbal part of our lives. It doesn't live in our conscious memory or persona, yet it can be the foundation of a person's ongoing experience. When we recognize it, we can address it somatically, for ourselves and our clients.

AN INTRIGUING PERSPECTIVE

Hubert began from this foundation on the first day of a workshop in Yverdon in 2011, the last of the series in Switzerland:

> Asking the question "What is a representation?" is the same as asking the question "What is perception?" Whether we say perception or representation, we are saying the same thing: because perception is not of "the real." Perception is representation. The raw material is already mediated.

A *representation* can be thought of as a pattern of neural activity that "stands in" for or maps certain features of the external or internal environment, allowing the brain to interpret, predict, and respond to sensory inputs and cognitive tasks. Perception is a representation in so far as it is not merely a passive recording of sensory information. Instead, it is an active, constructive process through which a person combines incoming sensory data with existing knowledge, memories, and expectations. The neuroscientist Ernst Kandel, who is known for his work on the biological basis of learning and memory, emphasizes that our perceptions are always partially filtered and interpreted, influenced by previous experience (see Chapter Fourteen). Neuroscientists may agree that perception is a construction, but for most of us that's an abstract concept, not our experience of daily life. To hear it put in such a matter-of-fact manner still reverberates with me to this day—"perception is not of the real."

For each one of us, the preverbal period of our lives is when this process of construction began.

Hubert painted an impressionist picture of this early stage of infancy for us:

The infant is an organism, bombarded by all forms of stimulation, making no distinction between the sensory modes. Auditory is not separate from tactile nor from sense of smell. The terms amodal—not linked to one sensory mode—or pluri-modal—all the modes together—express this quality of sensory experience. To create some "sense," some security from all this, the baby begins to extract covariants. For example, each time he hears the sound of someone speaking, he also sees their lips moving. An association begins to be created. This is an example of how perception is already a "representation," in the sense that it is made up of context and associations and is specific to the individual.

For most of us, seeing an infant brings an immediate response, based on the associations we have from our own past and our culture. When we meet a baby, we likely don't think of the objectified body—a baby is just too alive and responsive for that label. But putting all the associations aside, at the simplest level a baby is an organism embedded in an environment that includes the sensory world and the people they encounter. Both babies and adults are seeking—*not passively receiving*—and responding to sensory signals, streams of sensation, from within and without.

Hubert gave the example of a baby born prematurely who spends their first days in an incubator, where they will not be able to make an association between the sounds they hear and the movement of the lips of their caretaker. It doesn't mean that they can't catch up later on, he told us, but it shows how a random circumstance of the environment can impact the early development of perception/representation.

As adults, with our mental complexity, we lose sight and feel of the preverbal underpinnings of our own experience. I found it valuable that Hubert would keep bringing us back periodically to the developmental perspective, back to our beginnings, to how we begin to control our own movements, to when perception and anticipation begin.

WHAT NEWBORNS KNOW

Hubert's description resonated with my experience of encountering a newborn years before. The interesting research about babies' earliest interactions had made me very curious. I had not had the chance to observe this for myself as I had not borne children, so I was excited to get a call from my friend Richard on the day of his son Auren's birth. It was mid-morning, the baby had just been born, and we were invited to come meet him. He was the youngest human I had ever seen, let alone held.

In the hospital room, the blinds were open and bright light streamed in. Auren's eyes were tightly closed. Too bright for him, I thought. I lowered the blind, turning the louvers to lessen the brightness, while still allowing in some light. Right away, his eyelids opened, closed, opened, closed, as if his eyes were dancing with the light. The dimmer light invited a different interaction. He was already responding to his new surroundings, experimenting with movement and perception. With each movement of his eyes, associations were being established and practiced.

How does perception develop in infancy? From birth, and even somewhat before, there is a lot going on for a baby. Daniel Stern tells us that from day one,

> A baby's nervous system is prepared to evaluate immediately the intensity of a light, a sound, a touch—of anything accessible to one of his senses. How intensely he feels about something is probably the first clue he has available to tell him whether to approach it or to stay away. Intensity can lead him to try to protect himself. It can guide his attention and curiosity and determine his internal level of arousal. If something is only mildly intense (like a lamp lit in daylight), his attraction to it is weak. If too intense (like direct sunlight on him), he avoids it. But if it is moderately intense, like the patch of sunshine on the wall, he is spellbound. That just tolerable intensity and contrast arouses him. He immediately alters in response to it. It increases his animation, activates his whole being. (Stern, 1998, p.18)

The intensity has to be just the right amount. Too much, and the baby shuts down—just like Auren kept his eyes closed. At just the right level of stimulation, the baby responds with movement as a whole. The deep (tonic) muscles around his spine will arch his back; there will be wriggling, slower or faster kicking. All the musculature that will later become the scaffolding for reaching, sitting, standing, and walking is beginning to engage. But it isn't just a mechanical activity; it's a whole-system response, and as this chapter will explore, every experience for an infant has an emotional tone. A baby is no blank slate. Within hours of birth, they already begin the journey of organizing their experience of the world. With Auren, I had a role even in that brief moment: to pay attention to his signals and change the environment to support him.

EMOTION AND THE NEWBORN'S WORLD

"And all this is taking place in and with emotion. There is something we could call emotion that is a constant presence. The only thing that allows escape from this is representation," Hubert said.

The stream of sensations in which a baby lives is not just a sensory experience; it has emotional color. At the workshop in Yverdon, Hubert gave the example of a baby responding to their mother leaving the house. For the baby, at first when the mother leaves, she no longer exists. Imagine how terrifying that could feel! Once the baby has had enough opportunities to experience the mother's leaving and returning, they begin to have a sense of time and space. The mother's return becomes a possibility. The organization of memory based on experience gives the baby something to hang on to in the sea of sensation.

Hubert connected this aspect of infancy to our adult lives:

> In the beginning, every new movement is an emotion, and this may still be true for each of us as adults. So, when you ask why it is so hard to change—clearly, changing a gesture has an emotional dimension, just like for a newborn. It means to change the covariants, the basis of our security. But it is you who extracted that covariant, and it's you who is representing it. The covariant is not a fixed or given "reality."

Let's unpack Hubert's thinking. How is perception an emotional experience? What is a covariant? And what does all this have to do with our lives as adults or our ability to work with our movement patterns?

Although different authors may use these terms loosely, for the purposes of this book, we will use covariant to talk about what systematically moves together, a kind of coordination that ties together two elements—for example, gaze and head movement. As the head turns, the eyes adjust their position to stabilize the visual field. In a sense, the two parts have been linked neurologically, synaptically. By contrast, an invariant, like gravity, offers a reliable fixed point to expand the capacity of gesture. An invariant provides a reference upon which we can depend over time.

After a few weeks, baby Auren will begin to recognize patterns, sensory experiences that go together fairly consistently. This kind of sensory information begins to create order from chaos. Certain elements or aspects move together, appear together, like the body and the space. They are covariants. For example, as the hand moves, certain sensations accompany it and change in a regular way. Associations are forming, synapses are firing and wiring together. And with all this, gravity serves as a steady signal upon which to base the further elaboration of other gestures. While so many other things change, the signal of gravity is something to depend on—an invariant in the earthly domain.

The sensory information of covariance becomes a way to anticipate what will happen next—to predict—and that means to gain some control. During our first few months, our sense of body, our sense of self, is beginning to be assembled from sensory impressions that also form the background of our future emotions.

Meaning making has its beginning here, too: as sensations occur and reoccur, they become patterns, recognized and anticipated. Associations form. Perceptions begin to be selected and reinforced. Traces of our early movements, our first sense of embodiment, show up in the present. The first pre-movement patterns, patterns of perception—the very basis of emotional experience—it all starts here. As adults, the ability to experience real change in our own patterns sometimes has to reach this level, which is hard to access with our present consciousness because it comes before words.

Daniel Stern's book for parents, *Diary of a Baby: What Your Child Sees, Feels, and Experiences* (1998), charmingly combines the imagined journal entries of a baby, Joey, with explanations of early development that a layperson can understand. The evocative descriptions that follow expanded my understanding of the first few weeks of a baby's life in all its drama.

> Step into Joey's earliest world and recall what you have never really forgotten. Imagine that none of the things you see or touch or hear have names, and few [if] any memories attached to them. Joey experiences objects and events mainly in terms of feelings they evoke in him, and the opportunities for action they offer him. (Stern, 1998, p.13)

At six weeks, Stern places Joey in "the world of feelings." Not feelings such as "mad, sad, glad" but feelings at a much, much simpler level—levels of intensity that can attract or overwhelm. When his parents say his name, he doesn't know that the sound refers to him, or even that sound differs from touch. Yet a feeling tone is present: "He feels its glide, smooth and easy, soothing him; or its friction, turbulent and stirring him up, making him more alert" (Stern, 1998, p.13).

Stern captures the baby's experience and links it to our own. Imagine yourself as the news comes on your screen or radio. The tone of voice and the posture of the speaker are gliding over you the same way, stirring up your interest, your fears. As adults, our minds may be attending to other issues of past or future, but the same phenomena are communicating to us, and we are responding to them just as the baby would be.

THE WEATHERSCAPE

Stern describes Joey's experience as a "weatherscape": all the sensations and people and things are a seamless part of his experience. In our earliest days as a baby, we experience a flow of sensations without a sense of separation between inside and outside. Even Joey himself is an aspect of the weatherscape.

There are sensors in his skin for pressure, varied or enduring; hairs that allow him to detect stroking or friction. There are thermoreceptors that detect heat and cold, and nociceptors that detect pain. The information received by these sensors will combine with the sensory flows provided by the environment and eventually result in an interoceptive sense of self—the body image—and the kinesthetic/proprioceptive sense.

Bullinger, one of the experts in infant development introduced in Chapter Two, reminds us that proprioception isn't a physiological given, but a form of coordination between the receptors capturing information from the world, and the deep receptors embedded in the tissues, a construction made of smaller elements that can be combined in different ways (Bullinger, 2010, p.26). As Stern describes, at this point in a baby's life, in our own early lives, distinctions that we now take for granted do not exist—body, world, feelings, sensations—they are all part of the same weatherscape to which the baby belongs.

Separate vivid experiences exist. At six weeks, the baby still lives in a flow of sensory experiences, without words that make distinctions between sound, temperature, light. Without a clear sense of inside/outside. Stern calls this the emergent self (1985, pp.47ff.). What ties the experiences together into a coherent sense of self is yet to come.

> Like shots in a movie, one moment may be continuous with the next, or fade into it, or cut abruptly against it, or be separated from it by a blank

pause. It is not clear to Joey how he gets from one moment to the next, or what, if anything, happens between them. (Is it so clear for us?) But all his senses are focused on each one, and he lives each intensely. Many are the prototypes of moments that will recur over and over throughout his life. (Stern, 1998, p.15)

This is a baby's world at six weeks: dramatic and with no sense of control. Part of Stern's inquiry from the beginning of his research was to understand in what way a baby has a sense of self, "what kind of sense of self is possible during this initial period" (Stern, 1985, p.45)—still answering the initial question of what his patients are "remembering." At this time for Joey, there is no integration, or overarching "self." But there is the beginning of recognizing invariants and covariants, *always accompanying*.

As Hubert suggested, perception and emotion go together. Stern describes how, for Joey, just looking at the bars of his crib is a drama with feelings, excitement, thrill and fading.

[T]o Joey, the crib bar has certain abstract qualities: straightness; an elongated, thin shape; bright highlights, where the varnish reflects the light; high density; sharpness of form or outline against a more diffuse background; and so on. As each of these abstract qualities evokes a feeling in Joey, the bar provides an emotional experience. (Stern, 1998, p.26)

Have you ever thought of "emotional" in this way before? As adults, we imagine emotion as something much more complex. Recently, I was at a dinner party where a woman, a playwright, admitted that she didn't quite grasp the connection between emotions and the body. Another woman, a psychotherapist with an interest in trauma work, quickly answered that it was through associations: for instance, if someone yells at you when you are a child, your shoulders go up in a protective response. If it happens often enough, your shoulders might just stay up around your ears.

But I think Stern is leading us to see emotion at a much simpler and more foundational level: long before preschool, we are already responding to the intensity of sensory stimulation. Something arouses a response in us, we are drawn in or shy away, we wake up or calm down; at the simplest level, everything has a feeling tone. To Joey at six weeks, the simplest of moments, such as just lying in the crib with the sun on the bars, has a feeling—it is not just sensation alone, it is also an emotional experience. Perception and emotion are inseparable.

Even just feeling hungry—without being able to name or recognize hunger as such—is like a storm gathering. "The pulsing waves swell to dominate the whole weatherscape. The world is howling. Everything explodes and is blown out and then collapses and rushes back toward a knot of agony that cannot last—but does," Stern tells us (1998, p.32).

Imagine experiencing this level of intensity, six times a day! Joey doesn't know he is hungry. Stern's diary entry captures the storm of inchoate sensation that a baby might experience just in the course of every day. Stern calls these feelings "vitality affects": "surging, fading away, fleeting, explosive, crescendo, bursting, drawn out. These are forms of feeling that are connected with the vital processes of life" (Stern, 1985, p.54). They are the first building blocks of emotions.

Joey doesn't even know that he is crying. But his mother does. Along with the sound of his cry, his arousal or upset expresses itself as an arching of the back, kicking, or wriggling. There is an increase in muscular tone as part of the increase in intensity or feeling. In his developmental journey, the baby has no choice but to depend on other human beings for help. His human caretakers provide Joey's best way to manage the intense feelings that overtake him. When Joey's mother hears him crying with hunger, she comes over to the crib, picks him up, and holds him while she gets ready to breastfeed. Joey perceives vitality affects even in how he is picked up by his mom. Her touch will communicate with him.

TONIC DIALOGUE

Touch—all the signals coming from contact with surfaces and other people—is deeply tied into our body sense. Touch can stimulate a response from the most archaic movement system (spino-thalamic). The baby's body responds with an increase in tone. What Wallon described already beginning in utero, De Ajuriaguerra termed "tonic dialogue," the way the baby's body and the person holding the baby exchange through these primary movements (see Chapter Two). A deep emotional connection resonates through the sense of touch. This archaic system will never disappear but goes into the background of all our movements.

All the other sensory flows will travel through the same tonic mobilizations, a built-in repertory of responses. A stimulation presents itself and there will be a tonic response of contraction in the back muscles and then orienting toward the source. As the baby matures, his eyes, head, and chest will orient too. But for now, his mother's touch organizes Joey's physical experience. The way she supports him reassures him. The sound of her voice, the feeling of her touch, the movement and change in position are all contributing to creating an envelope that will embrace the child and help him change his state, his tonus. Wallon writes that "the baby belongs to the milieu before he belongs to himself" (quoted in Bullinger, 1998, p.33).

> She is talking to calm and reassure Joey (and also herself). What matters most is the music and the sound, not the lyrics. She uses the music of her voice as a blanket to wrap Joey in to soothe him, or at least to hold the fort for a moment until he starts to feed. She also uses her voice as a pacemaker, at first going faster than the beat of Joey's cries, to override his rhythm; then she slows down to bring him down with her to a less excited state. (Stern, 1998, pp.37–38)

The environment, including the caregiver, is part of what regulates tone for a baby (Bullinger, 1998, p.33). Stern describes what he calls "attuning," another talent infants use to make sense of their world. They can match the shapes, pacing, or intensity of their caretaker. And they can transfer the information between modes of sensory experience. Stern points out that there is a perceptual unity to sensory experience. The baby's representation of touch, vision, or sound can freely exchange independently of the specific channel. The term Stern uses for this capacity is "amodal perception" (Stern, 1985, p.51).

The simple act of being held upright is a dramatic change in tone for Joey. His mother's touch helps him feel contained, begins to shape a safe boundary. In addition to the comfort of the chest-to-chest connection, the vertical position (which Joey could not manage on his own) brings the baby into more relationship with the world around him.

> This vertical position is very special for young infants. The feedback from Joey's muscles tells him about his position in space and has a strong influence on the state of his nervous system. Putting a baby into the upright position is, for his nervous system, like switching gears in a car. He becomes quieted physically, but more alert mentally in the sense of being more open to the sights and sounds around him. (Stern, 1998, p.39)

This ordinary scene holds the key to essential aspects of our lives as adults, but they are hidden in plain sight. The sense of our own body's weight, the way we experience the space around us, the very way we perceive and respond to the constant flow of sensations, and the literal, physical support we receive that helps us shift states and organize tone are building blocks. They are the basis of our future movements. At this early age, a baby depends on someone else's body for soothing and managing the waves of sensation, but they are already forming associations that will carry through into adulthood.

As Hubert pointed out in his talk, relief from overwhelming sensations can come from a different relationship with the environment, a different experience of gravity, both in the young and in ourselves. At the earliest moment of development, some of the most important sensory information from the environment is directly from gravity. Gravity information comes through the two channels we have seen before: the vestibular system and the sense of weight.

At birth, we pass from a watery environment to an airy one, in which information is available in a very different way. Through tensions in the muscles, the infant feels the force that holds them to the ground when lying down. Gravity is experienced here as a sense of weight. In utero, there would be none of this kind of cue. In utero, only the signals from the vestibular system tell which way is up. Once a child is born, the two kinds of information accompany each other: the vestibular system's signals go along in a consistent way with the pressures induced by gravity on muscles, skin, and receptors.

Hubert said: "The only thing that is truly invariant in the world is gravity. Gravity is the only constant. Everything else changes all the time. Hence the importance of posture, emotion, space—it is all constructed in the same instant."

From our very first meeting, Hubert emphasized the importance of gravity as a consistent signal by which we can orient; and the way orientation, emotion, weight, and space are connected through our use of gravity. The European developmental perspective shows the starting point of so many patterns of movement, associations of meaning, and emotional experiences. While all this may live in a preverbal domain, working with a person in the present still includes all of them. Understanding these connections offers us many possibilities of change into adulthood.

MEETING AND RELATIONSHIP: THE PHYSICAL BASIS OF MEANING

Our physical experience as an infant provides our earliest conditioning. These building blocks include associations and meanings that form our future thoughts and feelings. Our sense of self, our sense of the surroundings, and our sense of other people all have a foundational relationship with the physical experience of being here, being together, that was built in our first year of life. This is part of the experience base that leads to a body that is "made not born."

Our caretaker's touch will communicate and shape the tone of our muscles. Experts such as Judith Kestenberg (mentioned in Chapter Two, Tonic function) have worked with the mother's way of holding their baby: a mismatch—too much tension or too little—and the baby learns to hold themselves, to create the missing relationship. In Didier Anzieu's idea of the "skin-ego" mentioned in Chapter Thirteen, the baby can use muscle tension to create an artificial skin when the sense of wholeness is lacking. This is also where *haptos* comes in—the way we begin to learn how to meet our surroundings, to be open to them, or defend from them. As adults, we may imagine that skin sensation and muscle tone are just physiological givens. But when we take the perspective of our development from infancy, we begin to understand the extent to which learning, selecting, and responding to early circumstances has shaped the body we know as "me."

Why is it so hard to change? While not every trouble we encounter throughout our childhood and adult lives has its roots in preverbal experience, imagining the developmental journey we have taken can be useful. To change a movement is often not a merely practical and pragmatic exercise. Our movement patterns offer security and protect us at a very primal level from the chaos we once experienced. Understanding the story of development—the way we have constructed security for ourselves—may help us meet the moments of unfamiliarity, the emotions that often accompany a perceptual shift, with less fear or at least with recognition that the moment of fear, rather than signaling something terrible, actually signals a new possibility. We can learn to welcome it.

Cradling Our Categories

THE BODY IS A NOMAD

The one thing we can all rely on is that we live in a world of change. For us to cultivate the sense of a reliable body, we need the skills to meet these changes without being thrown off balance. This quality of being is something we can practice through embodiment—which includes imagining. This is what building a reliable body requires.

At every stage of our ongoing development, we need to find a new equilibrium, a balance between old and new, independence and relatedness, a new movement possibility. At birth, the task is to construct a kinesphere, to "choose the good information" that can lead to stability in this moment without restricting our options. In aging, the task is how not to let our sense of space diminish, continuing to nourish the sense of weight along with the vestibular system, the inner ear, and the expanding horizon.

Throughout this book, we have explored different ways of conceptualizing, putting into words, and working with embodiment through practices, stories, and movement science. Many of the perspectives that Hubert introduced to us are reinforced on a daily basis by new research: individual movement signatures (Hug *et al.*, 2019) replace the idea of fixed muscle action; the homunculus now includes complex actions instead of cortical localization (Gordon *et al.*, 2023); the importance of pre-movement—the preparation *before* we act—is beginning to be recognized (Smoulder *et al.*, 2024). J. J. Gibson's understanding of affordances is used today to coach professional baseball players (Gray, 2024). What if we delighted in accepting that some of the categories we use today will be superseded by new discoveries, while some of our hunches will turn out to be true? Rather than clinging to our frameworks, we can cradle them, hold them gently, and be ready to let them go.

"The body is a nomad," Hubert said one day. "The body is always a variable, transitory, nomadic unfolding of a state of being, moment by moment" (Yverdon workshop, 2011). It reminded me of a scene from *Cave of Forgotten Dreams*, Werner Herzog's 2011 documentary about the Chauvet cave paintings. In the south of France, Chauvet is part of a dramatic landscape where limestone cliffs form an arch over the river Ardèche. Herzog and his team were allowed a rare opportunity to film inside the rock shelter where the cave paintings were discovered. Over 30,000 years old, the images of animal life depicted on the walls offer a glimpse of human experience from deep in prehistory.

These are action paintings: a group of lions stalks prey, all their eyes focused on something the viewer can't see; horses canter, buffalo surge. The images show close observation: the feathers of an owl, the movement of the horses' manes, the markings on a rhinoceros. The details suggest a close relationship between human and animal worlds that must have existed at that time. Yet the painters were not trying for accurate representation. As Herzog puts it, "the painters of Chauvet are not accountants of truth, of the variety of species... They are not cinema verité of their time" (Archaeology Magazine, 2011).

More than a thousand creatures appear on the walls of the Chauvet cave, but only one is a human figure. There is some mystery here: the image is wrapped around a stalactite and hard to discern. Is it a woman with the head of a bison, or a bison turning into a woman, or a woman transforming?

Herzog tells the interviewer, "Sometimes it is better to have a big question and no answer... It becomes much more an element that forces us to think, forces us to imagine, forces us to use all our intelligence and all our capacity for vision." Can we hold embodiment as a big question?

In Herzog's film, one of the curators tells the story of an ethnographer in northern Australia. Exploring with an Aboriginal guide, they arrived at a rock shelter with beautiful old paintings that were in decay. Seeing this, the guide felt moved to touch up the paintings, following the tradition of the area. When the ethnographer asked why he was painting, the man answered, "I am not painting, that's the hand spirit who is painting now. Because the man is a part of this spirit" (Herzog, 2011, 1:14:16–1:15:40). Like this Aboriginal guide, paleolithic people lived in a more fluid world, with categories that were cradled differently—an owl could become a man; a tree could speak; a woman could turn into a bison or vice versa. The curator in Herzog's film goes on to describe the permeability of the world of these ancient peoples in which a wall can talk to us, a wall can accept us or refuse us. The shaman could receive the visit of the supernatural or send the spirit out to roam. Permeable, fluid, shifting. It sounds familiar.

In our time, neuroscience provides remarkable imagery to invite us in the same direction as the cave paintings, towards a world with less defined boundaries. The body is a nomad. There is a kind of freedom, an openness to the imaginary, that is possible to approach even in this day and age. To feel comfortable with this freedom, this openness, requires an embodiment that reaches beyond repetition and identity. Coming back to orienting, being in an ongoing relationship with our surroundings based in artful, skillful managing of our instability, our relationship with gravity in this moment. Over the many years of working with Hubert, this theme was central, each time approached in a new way.

It was not until the last workshops in Cadiz (2015) that Hubert began to talk about ethics. Our haptic capacity, how we meet the world; our ability to find secure orientation without clinging to one position; to stand on our own while being able to accept the presence of the Other, these perspectives give an embodied dimension to a philosophy such as Martin Buber's (Buber, 1923/1996). Our stance, our gaze, can create a relationship of power or utility, *I–it*, where the other—or even our own body—is treated as an object to be used, analyzed, or manipulated. Or we can discover an *I–Thou* relationship. As an embodied experience, *I–Thou* is not merging, or a lack of stability or clarity. In practice, it is effective orientation, plus variability, adaptability, the ability to change our support that gives the confidence to be open, not to know. Cultivating a comfortable relationship with gravity, a recognition of this ongoing stream of information, helps our joints, helps our human relations, and helps our deepest longing for connection.

Works Cited

Alibert, M. (2014). *Yoga et santé énergétique*. Les Cahiers de Présence d'Esprit.

Allard, T., Clark, S. A., Jenkins, W. M., & Merzenich, M. M. (1991). Reorganization of somato-sensory area 3b representations in adult owl monkeys after digital syndactyly. *Journal of Neurophysiology*, *66*(3), 1048–1058. https://doi.org/10.1152/jn.1991.66.3.1048

Alpert, M. (2016). *The Six*. Sourcebooks Media Fusion.

Alpert, M. (n.d.). The science behind *The Six*. www.markalpert.com/books/the-six/science.php

Anzieu, D. (1995). *Le moi-peau*. Dunod.

Archaeology Magazine. (2011). Interview: Werner Herzog on the Birth of Art. *Archaeology Magazine*, *64*(2). https://archive.archaeology.org/1103/features/werner_herzog_chauvet_cave_forgotten_dreams.html

Bachelard, G., Farrell, E. R., & Farrell, C. F. (2011). *Air and Dreams: An Essay on the Imagination of Movement*. Dallas Institute Publications, Dallas Institute of Humanities and Culture.

Barrett, L. F. (2018). *How Emotions Are Made: The Secret Life of the Brain*. Houghton Mifflin Harcourt.

Bastian, H. C. (1887). The "muscular sense"; its nature and cortical localisation. *Brain*, *10*(1), 1–89. https://doi.org/10.1093/brain/10.1.1

BBC Horizon. (1998). *The Man Who Lost His Body* [Documentary film]. British Broadcasting Corporation. www.dailymotion.com/video/x12647t

Bernard, M. (2001). L'altérité originaire ou les mirages fondateurs de l'identité. *Protée*, *29*(3), 7–24. Quotes Wigman, M. (1986). *Le langage de la Danse*. Papiers.

Bernard, M. (2019). Sense and fiction, or the strange effects of three sensorial chiasms. hal-02292135. https://univ-paris8.hal.science/hal-02292135/document

Bernstein, N. (1967). *The Coordination and Regulation of Movements*. Pergamon Press.

Bertalanffy, L. von. (1952). *Problems of Life: An Evaluation of Modern Biological Thought*. Martino Fine Press.

Berthoz, A. (2000). *The Brain's Sense of Movement* (G. Weiss, trans.). Harvard University Press. (Original work published 1997)

Berthoz, A. (2012). *Simplexity: Simplifying Principles for a Complex World* (G. Weiss, trans.). Yale University Press. (Original work published 2009)

Berthoz, A. (2009). *La simplexité*. Odile Jacob.

Blakeslee, S., & Blakeslee, M. (2007). *The Body Has a Mind of Its Own: How Body Maps in Your Brain Help You Do (Almost) Everything Better*. Random House.

Body Worlds. (2024, May 29). Take an eye-opening journey under the skin! www.bodyworlds.com

Bolens, G. (2000). *La logique du corps articulaire: Les articulations du corps humain dans la littérature occidentale*. Presses Universitaires de Rennes.

Bolens, G. (2001). The limits of textuality: Mobility and fire production in Homer and Beowulf. *Oral Tradition*, *16*(1), 107–128. https://journal.oraltradition.org/wp-content/uploads/files/articles/16i/Bolens.pdf

Bonnier, P. (1900). *L'Orientation*. Carré & Naud.

Bordoni, B., Varacallo, M. A., Morabito, B., & Simonelli, M. (2019). Biotensegrity or fascintegrity? *Cureus*, *11*(6), e4819. https://doi.org/10.7759/cureus.4819

Buber, M. (1996). I and Thou (W. Kaufmann, trans.). Touchstone. (Original work published 1923)

Bull, N. (1968). *The Attitude Theory of Emotion*. Johnson Reprint Corporation. Retrieved from www.ibpj.org/issues/articles/Lewis%20-%20Nina%20Bull.pdf (Original work published 1951)

Bullinger, A. (1998). La genèse de l'axe corporel: Quelques repères. *Enfance*, *51*(1), 27–35.

Bullinger, A. (2010). *Le développement sensori-moteur de l'enfant et ses avatars*. Éditions érès.

CuriosityShow. (n.d.). Bumps and hollows illusion [Video]. YouTube. www.youtube.com/shorts/AZYYbQAxzio

Catani, M. (2017). A little man of some importance. *Brain*, *140*(11), 3055–3061. https://doi.org/10.1093/brain/awx270

Clark, S. A., Allard, T., Jenkins, W. M., & Merzenich, M. M. (1988). Receptive fields in the body-surface map in adult cortex defined by temporally correlated inputs. *Nature*, *332*(6163), 444–445. https://doi.org/10.1038/332444a0

Clemente, C. D. (1985). *Gray's Anatomy of the Human Body*. Lea & Febiger.

Cole, J. (1995). *Pride and a Daily Marathon*. MIT Press.

Collier, R. (2010). Cadaver shows stir controversy. *CMAJ*, *182*(14), E687–E688. https://doi.org/10.1503/cmaj.109-3351

Craig, A. B. (2015). *How Do You Feel?* Princeton University Press.

Creed, R. S., Sherrington, C. S., Denny-Brown, D., Eccles, J. C., & George, E. (1932). *Reflex Activity of the Spinal Cord*. Oxford University Press.

Cross, E. S., Liepelt, R., Hamilton, A. F., de C. Parkinson, J., Ramsey, R., Stadler, W., & Prinz, W. (2011). Robotic movement preferentially engages the action observation network. *Human Brain Mapping*, *33*(9), 2238–2254. https://doi.org/10.1002/hbm.21361

DARPAtv. (2015). DARPA Robotics Challenge 2015 Program Day02 [Video]. YouTube. www.youtube.com/watch?v=DkdESqML41g&list=PL6wMum5UsYvZuyGS54EFVMUdhaP4htD3F&index=6

De Beauvoir, S. (1956). *The Second Sex, Book II* (H. M. Parshley, trans.). Jonathan Cape. https://newuniversityinexileconsortium.org/wp-content/uploads/2021/07/Simone-de-Beauvoir-The-Second-Sex-Jonathan-Cape-1956.pdf (Original work published 1949)

Doidge, N. (2007). *The Brain that Changes Itself: Stories of Personal Triumph from the Frontiers of Brain Science*. Penguin Group.

Doidge, N. (2015). *The Brain's Way of Healing: Remarkable Discoveries and Recoveries from the Frontiers of Neuroplasticity*. Scribe Publications.

Dolto, F. (2014). *L'image inconsciente du corps*. Le Seuil.

Eagleman, D. (2020). *Livewired*. Doubleday Canada.

Edelman, G. M. (1992). *Bright Air, Brilliant Fire: On the Matter of the Mind*. Basic Books.

Fagenblat, M. (2017). *Negative Theology as Jewish Modernity*. Indiana University Press.

Feitis, R. (1978). *Ida Rolf Talks About Rolfing and Physical Reality*. The Rolf Institute.

Gallagher, S. (2005). *How the Body Shapes the Mind*. Oxford University Press.

Gallagher, S., & Cole, J. (2001). Body Image and Body Schema in a Deafferented Subject. In D. Welton (Ed.), *Body and Flesh: A Philosophical Reader* (pp.131–147). Blackwell Publishing. (Reprinted from "Body image and body schema in a deafferented subject," 1995, *The Journal of Mind and Behavior*, 16, pp.369–390.)

Gallese, V., Fadiga, L., Fogassi, L., & Rizzolatti, G. (1996). Action recognition in the premotor cortex. *Brain*, *119*, 593–609.

Gallese, V., & Sinigaglia, C. (2010). The bodily self as power for action. *Neuropsychologia*, *48*(3), 746–755. https://doi.org/10.1016/j.neuropsychologia.2009.09.038

Gallwey, W. T. (1974). *The Inner Game of Tennis: The Classic Guide to the Mental Side of Peak Performance*. Random House.

Gibson, J. J. (1966). *The Senses Considered as Perceptual Systems*. Houghton Mifflin.

Gibson, J. J. (1977). The Theory of Affordances. In R. Shaw & J. Bransford (Eds.), *Perceiving, Acting, and Knowing* (pp.67–82). Erlbaum Associates.

Godard, H., Amadori, D., & Bellani, M. (2001). Motion ed E-Motion in oncologia. *Manuale di Psiconologia* (pp.875–881). Masson.

Goldfield, E. (1995). *The Development of Action: A Dynamical Systems Approach*. MIT Press.

Gordon, E. M., Chauvin, R. J., Van, A. N., Rajesh, A., *et al.* (2023). A somato-cognitive action network alternates with effector regions in motor cortex. *Nature, 617*(7960), 351–359. https://doi.org/10.1038/s41586-023-05964-2

Gracovetsky, S. (1988). *The Spinal Engine*. Springer-Verlag.

Gracovetsky, S. (2007). *Stability or Controlled Instability*. In A. Vleeming (Ed.), *Movement, Stability, and Lumbopelvic Pain* (2nd ed., pp.279–293). Churchill Livingstone.

Gray, R. (2024). The Perception & Action Podcast. https://perceptionaction.com

Graziano, M. S. (2018). *The Spaces Between Us*. Oxford University Press.

Graziano, M. S., Taylor, C. S., & Moore, T. (2002). Complex movements evoked by microstimulation of precentral cortex. *Neuron, 34*, 841–851.

Grunwald, M. (2008). *Human Haptic Perception: Basics and Applications*. Birkhäuser.

Grunwald, M., & Weiss, T. (2005). Inducing sensory stimulation in the treatment of anorexia nervosa. *QJM: An International Journal of Medicine, 98*(5), 379–380. https://doi.org/10.1093/qjmed/hci061

Guggenheim Bilbao Museum. (n.d.). Walking Man I (Homme qui marche), 1960 [Teacher's Guide]. www.guggenheim-bilbao.eus/en/learn/schools/teachers-guides/walking-man-homme-qui-marche-1960

Gurfinkel, V. S. (1994). The mechanism of postural regulation in man. *Physiology and General Biology Reviews, 7*, 59–89.

Head, H., & Holmes, G. (1911). Sensory disturbances from cerebral lesions. *Brain, 34*, 102–254.

Head, H. (1926). *Aphasia and Kindred Disorders of Speech* (Vol. 1). Cambridge University Press.

Heglund, N., Willems, P., Penta, M., & Cavagna, G. (1995). Energy-saving gait mechanics with head-supported loads. *Nature, 375*(6526), 52–54. https://doi.org/10.1038/375052a0

Held, R., & Hein, A. (1963). Movement-produced stimulation in the development of visually guided behavior. *Journal of Comparative and Physiological Psychology, 56*(5), 872–876.

Herzog, W. (Director). (2011). *Cave of Forgotten Dreams* [Film]. IFC Films.

Hillman, J. (2021). Peaks and Vales: The Soul/Spirit Distinction as Basis for the Differences Between Psychotherapy and Spiritual Discipline. In G. Slater (Ed.), *Senex & Puer* (Vol. 3). Spring Publications. (Originally published in 1976.)

Holmes, N. P., & Spence, C. (2004). The body schema and the multisensory representation(s) of peripersonal space. *Cognitive Processing, 5*(2), 94–105. https://doi.org/10.1007/s10339-004-0013-3

Hug, F., Vogel, C., Tucker, K., Dorel, S., Deschamps, T., Le Carpentier, É., & Lacourpaille, L. (2019). Individuals have unique muscle activation signatures as revealed during gait and pedaling. *Journal of Applied Physiology, 127*(6), 1519–1529. https://doi.org/10.1152/japplphysiol.01101.2018

IEEE Spectrum. (2015). A Compilation of Robots Falling Down at the DARPA Robotics Challenge [Video]. YouTube. www.youtube.com/watch?v=g0TaYhjpOfo

indoContent. (2008). Monkey uses brain to control prosthetic arm [Video]. YouTube. www.youtube.com/watch?v=sm2dow87wQE

James, W. (1884). What is an emotion? *Mind, 9*(34), 188–205.

Jasanoff, A. (2018). *The Biological Mind: How Brain, Body, and Environment Collaborate to Make Us Who We Are*. Basic Books.

Jenkins, W. M., Merzenich, M. M., Ochs, M. T., Allard, T., & Guic-Robles, E. (1990). Functional reorganization of primary somatosensory cortex in adult owl monkeys after behaviorally controlled tactile stimulation. *Journal of Neurophysiology, 63*(1), 82–104. https://doi.org/10.1152/jn.1990.63.1.82

Johnson, D. (1995). *Bone, Breath, and Gesture*. North Atlantic Books.

Jostmann, N. B., Lakens, D., & Schubert, T. W. (2009). Weight as an embodiment of importance. *Psychological Science, 20*(9), 1169–1174. https://doi.org/10.1111/j.1467-9280.2009.02426.x

Kahn, J. (2010, November 8). The perfect stride. *The New Yorker*. www.newyorker.com/magazine/2010/11/08/the-perfect-stride

Kandel, E. R. (2006). *In Search of Memory: The Emergence of a New Science of Mind*. W. W. Norton & Company.

Kandel, E. R. (2016). *Reductionism in Art and Brain Science: Bridging the Two Cultures*. Columbia University Press.

Kashdan, T. B., Barrett, L. F., & McKnight, P. E. (2015). Unpacking emotion differentiation: Transforming unpleasant experience by perceiving distinctions in negativity. *Current Directions in Psychological Science, 24*(1), 10–16. https://doi.org/10.1177/0963721414550708

Kelso, J. A. S. (1982). *Human Motor Behavior: An Introduction*. Psychology Press.

Kelso, J. A. S. (1995). *Dynamic Patterns: The Self-Organization of Brain and Behavior*. The MIT Press.

Kleist, H. von. (1810). On the Marionette Theatre, The first of four parts. Source: Berliner Abendblatt No. 63 12.12.1810 [K. Keane, trans.] https://15orient.com/files/kleist-on-the-marionette-theatre.pdf

Kleist, H. von. (1810). On the Marionette Theatre, The second of four parts. Source: Berliner Abendblatt No. 64, 13.12.1810 [K. Keane, trans.] https://15orient.com/files/kleist-on-the-marionette-theatre.pdf

Körperwelten. (2024). Why are the plastinates posed the way they are? https://bodyworlds.com/exhibitions/human

Korzybski, A. (1933). *Science and Sanity: An Introduction to Non-Aristotelian Systems and General Semantics*. The International Non-Aristotelian Library Publishing Company.

Kuriyama, S. (2002). *The Expressiveness of the Body and the Divergence of Greek and Chinese Medicine*. Zone Books.

Kuypers, P. (2006). Des trous noirs: Un entretien avec Hubert Godard. *Nouvelles de Danse, 53,* 64–65. Éditions Contredanse.

Laban, R. von. (1966). *Choreutics: Annotated and edited by Lisa Ullmann*. Macdonald & Evans.

Lacan, J. (1966). *Écrits*. Le Seuil.

Lakoff, G. (2012). Explaining embodied cognition results. *Topics in Cognitive Science, 4*(4), 773–785. https://doi.org/10.1111/j.1756-8765.2012.01222.x

Lee, D. (1978). The Functions of Vision. In H. L. Pick & E. Saltzman (Eds.), *Modes of Perceiving and Processing Information*. Lawrence Erlbaum Associates.

Lee, J. (1946). *This Magic Body*. Viking Press.

Liepelt, R., Ullsperger, M., Obst, K., Spengler, S., von Cramon, D. Y., & Brass, M. (2009). Contextual movement constraints of others modulate motor preparation in the observer. *Neuropsychologia, 47*(1), 268–275.

Lishman, J. R., & Lee, D. N. (1973). The autonomy of visual kinaesthesis. *Perception, 2,* 287–294.

Llinás, R. (2002). *I of the Vortex*. MIT Press.

Lucas, G. (1977). *Star Wars IV: A New Hope*. [Film]. Twentieth Century Fox.

Maravita, A., & Iriki, A. (2004). Tools for the body (schema). *Trends in Cognitive Sciences, 8*(2), 79–86. https://doi.org/10.1016/j.tics.2003.12.008

Merleau-Ponty, M. (1964). *Le visible et l'invisible*. Gallimard.

Michaud, T. (1997). *Foot Orthoses and Other Forms of Conservative Foot Care*. Michaud.

Mickle, K. J., Munro, B. J., Lord, S. R., Menz, H. B., & Steele, J. R. (2009). Toe weakness and deformity increase the risk of falls in older people. *Clinical Biomechanics, 24,* 787–791.

Middendorf, I. (1990). *The Perceptible Breath: A Breathing Science*. Junfermann-Verlag.

MIT News. (1994, September 13). MIT's robotic fish takes first swim. Massachusetts Institute of Technology. https://news.mit.edu/1994/robotuna

Mulla, D. M., & Keir, P. J. (2023). Neuromuscular control: From a biomechanist's perspective. *Frontiers in Sports and Active Living, 5,* 1217009. https://doi.org/10.3389/fspor.2023.1217009

Napier, J. R. (1967). The antiquity of human walking. *Scientific American, 216,* 55–66.

Nashner, L. M., & Cordo, P. J. (1981). Relation of automatic postural responses and reaction-time voluntary movements of human leg muscles. *Experimental Brain Research, 43*(3–4), 395–405. https://doi.org/10.1007/BF00238382

Nasio, J. D. (2007). *Mon corps et ses images*. Payot.

Newton, A. (2011). Stabilization: The Core and Beyond. In E. Dalton (Ed.), *Dynamic Body*. Freedom From Pain Institute. https://alinenewton.com/the-physical-intelligence-initiative

NHL Overtimes. (2021, August 10). 1988 Olympics 100m semi-finals: Ben Johnson, Carl Lewis [Video]. YouTube. www.youtube.com/watch?v=Wcya6ccGfVg

Nike. (1988, July 1). Just Do It [Advertisement].

Orbach, S. (1979). *Fat Is a Feminist Issue*. Berkley Books.

Orbach, S. (2009). *Bodies*. Profile Books.

Paillard, J. (1999). Body Schema and Body Image: A Double Dissociation in Deafferented Patients. In G. N. Gantchev, S. Mori, & J. Massion (Eds.), *Motor Control Today and Tomorrow* (pp.197–214). Academic Publishing House. http://espra.scicog.fr/PAILLARD%20269%20Body%20schema%20Image%20Deaf%201999.pdf

Paillard, J. (2005) 'Vectorial versus Configural Encoding of Body Space, A neural basis for a distinction between Body schema and Body image.' In : V.Knockaert & H. De Preester (eds) *Body Image and Body Schema: Interdisciplinary perspectives*. Amsterdam:John Benjamin.

Palmer, W. (1999). *The Intuitive Body*. North Atlantic Books.

Penfield, W., & Boldrey, E. (1937). Somatic motor and sensory representation in the cerebral cortex of man as studied by electrical stimulation. *Brain*, *60*, 389–440.

Pfeifer, R., & Bongard, J. (2007). *How the Body Shapes the Way We Think: A New View of Intelligence*. MIT Press.

Proske, U., & Gandevia, S. C. (2009). The kinaesthetic senses. *The Journal of Physiology*, *587*(17), 4139–4146. https://doi.org/10.1113/jphysiol.2009.175372

Rabellino, D., Frewen, P. A., McKinnon, M. C., & Lanius, R. A. (2020). Peripersonal space and bodily self-consciousness: Implications for psychological trauma-related disorders. *Frontiers in Neuroscience*, *14*. https://doi.org/10.3389/fnins.2020.586605

Ramachandran, V. S. (1994). Phantom limbs, neglect syndromes, repressed memories, and Freudian psychology. *International Review of Neurobiology*, *37*, 291–333. https://doi.org/10.1016/S0074-7742(08)60254-8

Reed, E. S. (1982). An outline of a theory of action systems. *Journal of Motor Behavior*, *14*(2), 98–134. https://doi.org/10.1080/00222895.1982.10735267

Reed, E. S. (1988). *James J. Gibson and the Psychology of Perception*. Yale University Press.

Reed, E. S. (1996). *Encountering the World: Toward an Ecological Psychology*. Oxford University Press.

Ribot-Ciscar, E., Rossi-Durand, C., & Roll, J. P. (2000). Increased muscle spindle sensitivity to movement during reinforcement maneuvers in relaxed human subjects. *The Journal of Physiology*, *523*(Pt 1), 271–282.

Rolf, I. (1977). *Rolfing: The Integration of Human Structures*. Dennis-Landman Publishers.

Ross, D. F., Read, J. D., & Toglia, M. (1994). *Adult Eyewitness Testimony: Current Trends and Developments*. Cambridge University Press.

Sachs, J. (n.d.). Aristotle: Poetics. Internet Encyclopedia of Philosophy. https://iep.utm.edu/aristotle-poetics

Salomon, R., Ronchi, R., Dönz, J., Bello-Ruiz, J., *et al.* (2016). The insula mediates access to awareness of visual stimuli presented synchronously to the heartbeat. *The Journal of Neuroscience*, *36*(18), 5115–5127. https://doi.org/10.1523/JNEUROSCI.4262-15.2016

Sattin, D., Parma, C., Lunetta, C., Zulueta, A., et al. (2023). An overview of the body schema and body image: Theoretical models, methodological settings, and pitfalls for rehabilitation of persons with neurological disorders. *Brain Sciences*, *13*(10), 1410. https://doi.org/10.3390/brainsci13101410

Schmidt, M. (2009, May 31). Hips are bringing more athletes to their knees. *The New York Times*. www.nytimes.com/2009/06/01/sports/01hips.html

Schmitz, T., De Rosa, E., & Anderson, A. (2009). Opposing influences of affective state valence on visual cortical encoding. *The Journal of Neuroscience*, *29*(22), 7199–7207.

Schwarzlose, R. (2021). *Brainscapes*. Houghton Mifflin Harcourt.

Science News. (2008, May 28). Monkey think, robotic monkey arm do. www.sciencenews.org/article/monkey-think-robotic-monkey-arm-do

Sherrington, C. S. (1931). Quantitative management of contraction in lowest-level coordination (Hughlings Jackson Lecture). *Brain*, *54*, 1–28.

Shumway-Cook, A., Woollacott, M. H., Rachwani, J., & Santamaria, V. (2024). *Motor Control*. Lippincott Williams & Wilkins.

Smoulder, A. L., Marino, P. J., Oby, E. R., Snyder, S. E., *et al.* (2024). A neural basis of choking under pressure. *Neuron, 112*(20), 3424–3433. https://doi.org/10.1016/j.neuron.2024.08.012

Sohier, R., & Haye, M. (1989). *Deux marches pour la machine humaine*. Éditions Kiné-Sciences.

Spencer, J., Clearfield, M., Corbetta, D., Ulrich, B., Buchanan, P., & Schöner, G. (2006). Moving toward a grand theory of development: In memory of Esther Thelen. *Child Development, 77*(6), 1521–1538. https://dynamicfieldtheory.org/upload/file/1553697968_87343ea4076733ecbfa0/Spencer_PublishedVersion2006.pdf

Spiers, H. J., & Maguire, E. A. (2007). Neural substrates of driving behaviour. *NeuroImage, 36*(1), 245–255. https://doi.org/10.1016/j.neuroimage.2007.02.032

Standring, S. (2008). *Gray's Anatomy: The Anatomical Basis of Clinical Practice* (40th ed.). Elsevier Churchill Livingston.

Stebbins, G. (1885). *The Delsarte System of Dramatic Expression*. Edgar S. Werner.

Stern, D. (1985). *The Interpersonal World of the Infant: A View from Psychoanalysis and Developmental Psychology*. Basic Books.

Stern, D. (1998). *Diary of a Baby: What Your Child Sees, Feels, and Experiences*. Basic Books.

Stoffregen, T. A., & Riccio, G. E. (1988). An ecological theory of orientation and the vestibular system. *Psychological Review, 95*(1), 3–14. https://doi.org/10.1037/0033-295X.95.1.3

Stuart, D. G. (2005). Integration of posture and movement: Contributions of Sherrington, Hess, and Bernstein. *Human Movement Science, 24*(5–6), 621–643. https://doi.org/10.1016/j.humov.2005.09.011

TheCoach. (2012). The Inner Game of Tennis. [Video]. YouTube. www.youtube.com/watch?v=-gowpi5ipNE

Thelen, E. (1998). The Improvising Infant: Learning About Learning to Move. In J. S. DeLoache, S. C. Mangelsdorf, & E. Pomerantz (Eds.), *Current Readings in Child Development* (3rd ed., pp.26–42). Allyn and Bacon.

Thelen, E. (2005). Dynamic systems theory and the complexity of change. *Psychoanalytic Dialogues, 15*(2), 255–283. https://doi.org/10.1080/10481881509348831

Thelen, E., & Smith, L. B. (1995). *A Dynamic Systems Approach to the Development of Cognition and Action*. MIT Press.

Tobias, P. V. (1982). *Man, the Tottering Biped: The Evolution of His Posture, Poise, and Skill*. University of New South Wales.

Triantafyllou, M. S., & Triantafyllou, G. S. (1995). An efficient swimming machine. *Scientific American, 272*(3), 64–70.

Ungerleider, L. G., & Mishkin, M. (1982). Two Cortical Visual Systems. In D. J. Ingle, M. A. Goodale, & R. J. Mansfield (Eds.), *Analysis of Visual Behavior* (pp.549–586). MIT Press.

Velliste, M., Perel, S., Spalding, M. C., Whitford, A. S., & Schwartz, A. B. (2008). Cortical control of a prosthetic arm for self-feeding. *Nature, 453*(7198), 1098–1101. https://doi.org/10.1038/nature06996

Wallon, H. (1956). Importance du mouvement dans le développement psychologique de l'enfant. *Enfance, 9*(2), 1–4. https://doi.org/10.3406/enfan.1956.1508

Warner Bros. Classics. (2016, October 24). The Babbit and the Bromide—Fred Astaire and Gene Kelly | Ziegfeld Follies | Warner Archive [Video]. YouTube. www.youtube.com/watch?v=c1GV5o5xNqU

Watts, A. (n.d.). The nature of consciousness [Lecture transcript]. Awaken. www.awaken.com/alan-watts-the-nature-of-consciousness

Weiner, N. (1950). *The Human Use of Human Beings: Cybernetics and Society*. Houghton-Mifflin.

Weiskrantz, L., Warrington, E. K., Sanders, M. D., & Marshall, J. (1974). Visual capacity in the hemianopic field following a restricted occipital ablation. *Brain, 97*(1), 709–728. https://doi.org/10.1093/brain/97.1.709

Weiskrantz, L. (1989). Blindsight. In F. Boller, & J. Grafman (Eds.), *Handbook of Neuropsychology* (Vol. 2, pp.375–385). Elsevier.

Wiesendanger, M. (1984). Pyramidal tract function and the clinical "pyramidal syndrome". *Human Neurobiology, 2*(4), 227–234.

Wigman, M. (1986). *Le langage de la danse*. Éditions Papier.

Wilhelm, R., Baynes, C. F., Jung, C. G., & Wilhelm, H. (1967). *The I Ching or Book of Changes*. Princeton University Press.

Wilson, F. (1999). *The Hand*. Vintage Books.

Winnicott, D. W. (1953). Transitional objects and transitional phenomena: A study of the first not-me possession. *The International Journal of Psychoanalysis*, 34, 89–97.

World Health Organization. (2021). Falls. www.who.int/news-room/fact-sheets/detail/falls

YAMAX. (n.d.). About us. www.yamax-yamasa.com/aboutus

Yeh, T. T., Cluff, T., & Balasubramaniam, R. (2014). Visual reliance for balance control in older adults persists when visual information is disrupted by artificial feedback delays. *PLoS ONE*, 9(3), e91554. https://doi.org/10.1371/journal.pone.0091554

Yong, E. (2022). *An Immense World: How Animal Senses Reveal the Hidden Realms Around Us*. Penguin Random House.

Young, I. M. (1980). Throwing like a girl: A phenomenology of feminine body comportment, motility, and spatiality. *Human Studies*, 3, 137–156.

Endnotes

Introduction
1   Rolfing®, Rolfer®, and Rolf Movement® are service marks of The Rolf Institute of Structural Integration®, Boulder, CO.
2   Françoise Mézieres (1909–1991) was a French physiotherapist who developed a method of global postural re-education.
3   For an in-depth description of Hubert's approach to core and how it differs from the standard, see Newton, A. (2011). Stabilization: The Core and Beyond. In E. Dalton (ed.). *Dynamic Body*. Freedom From Pain Institute. https://alinenewton.com/stabilization-the-core-and-beyond

Chapter 1
1   As Edward Reed, Gibson's biographer, explains in "Orientation to gravity is, in fact, something of a misnomer, as what needs to be regulated is the potentially disorienting effects of an animal's actions within a field of forces conditioned by gravity (Stoffregen & Riccio, 1988, p.88).
2   Alfred Korzybski (1879–1950) was a Polish American scholar who developed the field of General Semantics.
3   Sensitive dependence on initial conditions, another tenet of a dynamic systems approach.
4   Moshe Feldenkrais (1904–1984) was a somatic pioneer, and a contemporary of Dr. Rolf.

Chapter 2
1   We are using center of gravity and center of mass synonymously here. Technically, the center of gravity is the vertical projection of the center of the mass of the whole body.
2   The stretch reflex.
3   There isn't necessarily a great definition of tone, but let's go with "the overall stiffness of the muscle" or resistance to stretch: "The more usual definition of tone refers to muscular readiness to respond to nervous stimuli. J. V. Basmajian calls attention to the factor of tissue resilience as a significant part of tone" (Rolf, 1977, p.39).

Chapter 3
1   For an analysis of the walking vs running debate, see https://en.wikipedia.org/wiki/Endurance_running_hypothesis
2   This perspective differs from L. F. Barrett's. She says the brain evolved to oversee our internal systems. Both are surely partially true, but the sea squirt suggests that if you don't circulate in the world, you don't need a brain. For contrasting views, see Llinás (2002); Barrett (2018).
3   The technical term for vision's ability to zoom in and out is "vergence."
4   Stiff orthotics don't allow for the natural movement of the joints (the talus and tibia), which can lead to knee problems (Michaud, 1997).

Chapter 4

1   Hubert credits F. M. Alexander as an important influence in orienting his own approach to movement. F. M. Alexander used the terms "means whereby" for the attention to the process, and "end-gaining as a pejorative term for disregarding the means in favor of the goal."

Chapter 5

1   When I heard this from my client, I wondered what partial understanding it evolved from: I think perhaps the teacher was looking for the trapezius muscles not to work first. But far from not moving at all, for shoulders to keep their biomechanical integrity, the scapula has to adapt as the arm comes up to change the orientation of the acromion to allow the meeting of humerus and scapula.

Chapter 6

1   For a good summary of Gibson's use of affordance, see Blakeslee, S., & Blakeslee, M. (2007). *The Body Has a Mind of Its Own: How Body Maps in Your Brain Help You Do (Almost) Everything Better.* Random House, pp.105–108.
2   Students in a dance program have told me: "I don't feel my body unless it hurts."

Chapter 7

1   The quote is my paraphrase. The first of four parts. Source: Berliner Abendblatt No. 63 12.12.1810, Translated by Kevin J. M. Keane, https://15orient.com/files/kleist-on-the-marionette-theatre.pdf
2   The second of four parts. Source: Berliner Abendblatt No. 64, 13.12.1810.

Chapter 8

1   Alain Berthoz (b. 1939), Emeritus Professor at the Collège de France and Director of the Laboratory of Physiology of Perception and Action at the Centre National de la Recherche Scientifique (CNRS).
2   See Tobias, 1982 for the evolutionary perspective—a discussion about primate evolution organizing sitting and reaching before standing.

Chapter 9

1   Don Miller: https://mastodontaichi.com
2   Free flow and bound flow are the choreographer and dance theorist Rudolf von Laban's (1879–1958) terms. See https://en.wikipedia.org/wiki/Laban_movement_analysis

Chapter 10

1   In addition to the article by Gallagher and Cole, Ian Waterman's story is told by one of the authors of the paper (Cole) in the biography *Pride and a Daily Marathon* (1995) and the film *The Man Who Lost His Body* (BBC Horizon, 1998).
2   Peripheral nerves are large fibers covered in an insulating sheath of myelin, a fatty layer that speeds up transmission of electrical signals.
3   The terms kinesthesis, kinesthesia, and kinesthetic sense are used synonymously in this text.
4   "Myelin is an insulating layer, or sheath that forms around nerves, including those in the brain and spinal cord. It is made up of protein and fatty substances. This myelin sheath allows electrical impulses to transmit quickly and efficiently along the nerve cells." https://medlineplus.gov/ency/article/002261.htm

Chapter 11

1   These two kinds of information were described in Gibson, 1966.
2   Berthoz gives examples of active movement inhibiting tactile perception; of some neurons in the superior temporal sulcus stopping their firing when the animal's arm comes into view: "These effects are not due to the simple fact of attention. They are actually very

selective inhibitions of an aggregate of multisensory properties (texture, visual aspect, space) of a part of the body of a monkey or a known object. Perception is selection and anticipation. Time will reveal their mechanism" (Berthoz, 2000, p.88).

Chapter 12
1   As depicted in the film *The Man Who Lost His Body* (BBC Horizon, 1998, 42:06, 48:29–48:30; British Broadcasting Corporation. www.dailymotion.com/video/x12647t)
2   For a detailed description of dogs' sense of smell, see Yong, E. (2022). *An Immense World, How Animal Senses Reveal the Hidden Realms Around Us.* Penguin Random House, pp.17–26.

Chapter 13
1   For a good description of how skin signals become representations, see Schwarzlose, R. (2021). *Brainscapes.* Houghton Mifflin Harcourt, pp.10–14; for a discussion of the debate between theories of representation and enaction, see: https://en.wikipedia.org/wiki/Enactivism
2   Using receptors in the skin that respond to pain or temperature as well as the free nerve endings that are sensitive to pain, temperature, and muscle fatigue.
3   Ramachandran is the researcher who did the experiments on phantom limbs mentioned in the Introduction. www.edge.org/documents/Rama-2000.pdf

Chapter 14
1   V1 for vision; lateral occipital cortex for visual-tactile, and amygdala, hypothalamus, insula, dopaminergic pathways for signals that stir emotion.
2   See Newton, 2011.
3   Sometimes Hubert used the French term "semi-fixe" (i.e., partially fixed) to prevent us from creating unnecessary tension trying to "fixate." The two points could be moving away from each other also.
4   A vector is a quantity that has both magnitude and direction, but not position. www.britannica.com/science/vector-physics
5   See previous section, *Non-doing*; Hubert called the change in what moves and what stays still "changing the fixed point."
6   Buddha in Lankavatara Sutra states, "Things are not what they seem... Deeds exist, but no doer can be found" (Majjhima Nikaya, 192).
7   Eastern imagination did not create the same separation. See Kuriyama, 2002.

Chapter 15
1   "Sense of agency (the sense of being the one who generates an action) and/or sense of ownership (the sense of being the one who undergoes any experience, no matter if internally or externally generated)" (Gallese & Sinigaglia, 2010).
2   Kinesphere: "the sphere around the body whose periphery can be reached by easily extended limbs without stepping away from that place which is the point of support when standing on one foot, which we shall call the 'stance'" (Laban, 1966, p.10)
3   "Peripersonal space (PPS) is defined as the space surrounding the body where we can reach or be reached by external entities, including objects or other individuals." PPS is an essential component of bodily self-consciousness that allows us to perform actions in the world (e.g., grasping and manipulating objects) and protect our body while interacting with the surrounding environment (Rabellino et al., 2020)
4   See Wilson, F. (1999). *The Hand.* Vintage Books, pp.63–66 for a great description of crane operating.
5   *Rogue One: A Star Wars Story* (2016), directed by Gareth Edwards, produced by Lucasfilm.
6   Attributed to Huineng the Sixth, Patriarch of the Chan (Zen) school of Buddhism.

Chapter 16
1   Gemma Martino was the director of the Pain and Rehabilitation department at Istituto Nazionale dei Tumori, and collaborated with Hubert for many years.

2   Electromyography (EMG) measures and records skeletal muscle's electrical activity.
3   Gamma motor neurons (also known as γ-motoneurones) increase the sensitivity of the muscle spindles to stretch. With the alpha motor neurons (also known as α-motoneurones), they are important components of the stretch reflex. For a more nuanced understanding, see Ribot-Ciscar *et al.,* (2000, p.271): "Whereas in amphibia, terminal branches of α-motoneurones provide motor innervation to muscle spindles, in mammals, a separate fusimotor supply has evolved, namely γ-motoneurones. These are morphologically different from α-motoneurones, they receive different reflex connections, and they innervate muscle spindles separately and more extensively. Together this suggests that the fusimotor system might, to some extent, act independently of the skeletomotor system and could modify muscle spindle sensitivity selectively in order to make the receptors extract more accurate information movement."
4   G' describes a partial center of gravity seen from the middle of the chest around T4 in reference to the transverse axis connecting the two heads of femurs. See Chapter Eight.

Chapter 17
1   Look back at Chapter One, Esther Thelen's work, and the Dynamic Systems approach to embodiment.
2   Gerda Alexander (1908–1994), German/Danish somatic pioneer. See Johnson, D. (1995). *Bone, Breath, and Gesture.* North Atlantic Books, Chapter Three, pp.253–294.
3   Sometimes translated as "Ba Bei-han Xiong"—raise back, hollow chest—and may be offered in a different order (hollow the front and expand the back), depending on the school.
4   Translation mine.

Index